Psychiatry

NOTICE

Medicine is an ever-changing science. As new research and clinical experience broaden our knowledge, changes in treatment and drug therapy are required. The editors and the publisher of this work have checked with sources believed to be reliable in their efforts to provide information that is complete and generally in accord with the standards accepted at the time of publication. However, in view of the possibility of human error or changes in medical sciences, neither the editors, nor the publisher, nor any other party who has been involved in the preparation or publication of this work warrants that the information contained herein is in every respect accurate or complete. Readers are encouraged to confirm the information contained herein with other sources. For example and in particular, readers are advised to check the product information sheet included in the package of each drug they plan to administer to be certain that the information contained in this book is accurate and that changes have not been made in the recommended dose or in the contraindications for administration. This recommendation is of particular importance in connection with new or infrequently used drugs.

Psychiatry

PreTest® Self-Assessment and Review

Fifth Edition

Edited by

Sherwyn M. Woods, M.D., Ph.D.
Professor of Psychiatry
Director, Student Psychiatric Services
Director, Psychoanalytic Education
University of Southern California School of Medicine
Los Angeles County / USC Medical Center
Los Angeles, California

McGraw-Hill Information Services Company
Health Professions Division
PreTest Series

*New York St. Louis San Francisco Colorado Springs Auckland Bogotá Hamburg
Lisbon London Madrid Mexico Milan Montreal New Delhi Panama Paris
San Juan São Paulo Singapore Sydney Tokyo Toronto*

Library of Congress Cataloging-in-Publication Data

Psychiatry : PreTest self-assessment and review / edited by Sherwyn M.
  Woods.—5th ed.
    p.   cm.
    Bibliography: p.
    ISBN 0-07-051970-6 : $14.95
    1. Psychiatry—Examinations, questions, etc. 2. Woods, Sherwyn M.
    [DNLM: 1. Psychiatry—examination questions. WM 18 P978]
  RC457.P78   1989
  616.89′0076—dc19
  DNLM/DLC
  for Library of Congress   89-2730
                                                                      CIP

This book was set in Times Roman by Waldman Graphics, Inc.; the editors
were J. Dereck Jeffers and Bruce MacGregor; the production supervisor was
Clara B. Stanley.
R. R. Donnelley & Sons was printer and binder.

1 2 3 4 5 6 7 8 9 0   DOCDOC   8 9 4 3 2 1 0 9

ISBN 0-07-051970-6

Contents

Preface

This fifth edition of *Psychiatry, PreTest Self-Assessment and Review* has been extensively redesigned and revised. The chapters have been newly titled and reorganized, new chapters have been added, and the field of psychiatry has been covered in greater depth and breadth. The questions and explanations are now consistent with the terminology and definitions employed by the revised third edition of the *Diagnostic and Statistical Manual of Mental Disorders* of the American Psychiatric Association. The references have been updated, and all questions are now referenced to standard textbooks and major resource books that are readily available in most libraries.

I would like to express special gratitude to my wife, Nancy Bricard Woods, for her encouragement, patience, and support. I am also deeply appreciative of the assistance of all those who were so helpful in the preparation of this manuscript, including Mary Jane Costello, Charles Patterson, M.D., Edmond Pi, M.D., and Warner Johnson, M.D.

Sherwyn M. Woods, M.D., Ph.D.

Introduction

Psychiatry, PreTest Self-Assessment and Review, 5th Ed., has been designed to provide medical students, psychiatric residents, psychiatrists, and mental health professionals with a comprehensive and convenient instrument for self-assessment and review within the field of psychiatry. The 500 questions provided have been designed to parallel the topics, format, and degree of difficulty of the questions contained in Part II of the National Board of Medical Examiners examinations, the Federation Licensing Examination (FLEX), and the Foreign Medical Graduate Examination in the Medical Sciences (FMGEMS). The questions are also of a style and variety that should prove useful to those preparing for the certification examinations of the American Board of Psychiatry and Neurology.

Each question in the book is accompanied by an answer, a paragraph explanation, and a specific page reference to a textbook or major resource. These reference sources have been carefully selected for their educational excellence and ready availability in most libraries. A bibliography that lists all the sources used in the book follows the last chapter.

One effective way to use this book is to allow yourself one minute to answer each question in a given chapter; as you proceed, indicate your answer beside each question. By following this suggestion, you will be approximating the time limits imposed by the board examinations previously mentioned.

Since there are few absolutes in clinical practice, remember to simply choose the best possible answer. There are no "trick" questions intended. Rather, each has been designed to address a significant topic. All questions apply to the evaluation and treatment of adults, unless children or adolescents are specifically mentioned.

When you have finished answering the questions in a chapter, you should then spend as much time as you need verifying your answers and carefully reading the explanations. Although you should pay special attention to the explanations for the questions you answered incorrectly, you should read every explanation. The author of this book has designed the explanations to reinforce and supplement the information tested by the questions. If, after reading the explanations for a given chapter, you feel you need still more information about the material covered, you should consult and study the references indicated.

Psychiatry

Evaluation, Assessment, and Diagnosis

DIRECTIONS: Each question below contains five suggested responses. Select the **one best** response to each question.

1. The most frequent indication for psychological testing in clinical psychiatry is

(A) to determine the correct dosage of medication
(B) to determine the most effective psychotherapeutic style
(C) to assist when there is uncertainty about the diagnosis
(D) to assist in determining the length of treatment
(E) to assist in generating clinical impressions

2. Brain-imaging techniques, such as computed tomography (CT), would be most useful in evaluating

(A) bipolar disorder
(B) schizophrenia
(C) panic disorder
(D) Alzheimer dementia
(E) sleep apnea

3. All the following are projective tests EXCEPT

(A) Rorschach
(B) thematic apperception test
(C) Zung
(D) draw a human figure
(E) sentence completion

4. The intelligence quotient (IQ) is best described as a measure of

(A) innate cognitive endowment
(B) future cognitive potential
(C) environmentally determined cognitive skill
(D) present functional cognitive ability
(E) learned verbal skills

5. Determination of the urinary concentration of 3-methoxy-4-hydroxyphenylglycol (MHPG) may be helpful in which of the following clinical situations?

(A) Differentiating acute from chronic schizophrenia
(B) Distinguishing subtypes of primary affective disorder
(C) Predicting which hypertensive persons will develop depression as a complication of reserpine therapy
(D) Choosing antidepressant therapy for persons with unipolar depression
(E) Evaluating sleep disturbances

6. In the United States, the sex ratio (female-to-male) of successful suicides is approximately

(A) 4:1
(B) 2:1
(C) 1:1
(D) 1:3
(E) 1:6

7. A delusion can best be defined as a

(A) false belief that meets specific psychological needs
(B) perceptual misrepresentation of a sensory image
(C) perceptual representation of a sound or object not actually present
(D) viewpoint able to be changed when convincing evidence to the contrary is presented
(E) dissociative reaction

8. A 7-year-old girl hospitalized for a tonsillectomy awakens and cries out in fright that a "big bear" is in her room. She is relieved when a nurse, responding to her cry, enters the room and turns on the light, revealing the bear to be an armchair covered with a coat. This experience would be an example of

(A) a delusion
(B) a hallucination
(C) an illusion
(D) déjà vu
(E) dissociative reaction

9. In assessing the contribution of genetic factors in a psychiatric disorder, the psychiatrist

(A) asks the patient to report a recent dream
(B) reviews the psychosexual history
(C) collects information about the psychiatric hospitalization of relatives
(D) takes a blood sample for a complete blood count
(E) requests psychological testing

10. Persons who ultimately commit suicide are most likely to be

(A) secretive about their intent
(B) reluctant to seek help from physicians
(C) orderly and controlling in their personality style
(D) a member of a family with a history of suicide
(E) psychotic

11. Calculation of an IQ score requires knowledge of an examinee's

(A) mental age and educational level
(B) chronological age and educational level
(C) mental age and chronological age
(D) mental age, chronological age, and educational level
(E) mental age and psychiatric history

12. Suicide risk is lowest among people who are

(A) single
(B) married
(C) separated
(D) divorced
(E) widowed

13. An 18-year-old woman, previously in good health, seeks help at an emergency room for lightheadedness, headaches, and nausea. She appears anxious and is tremulous, sweating, and breathing heavily. While waiting to see a physician, she begins to complain of tingling around her mouth and in her fingertips. The physician should first

(A) ask her to breathe into a paper bag
(B) order immediate intravenous infusion of 50 ml of 50% glucose solution
(C) arrange for a brain scan
(D) conduct an amobarbital interview
(E) draw a blood sample to evaluate blood alcohol concentration

14. As part of a mental status examination, an interviewer asks,"What is the similarity between a chair and a table?" The interviewee replies, "They both have legs." This response is an example of

(A) abstract thinking
(B) concrete thinking
(C) bizarre thinking
(D) idiosyncratic thinking
(E) a passive-aggressive personality

15. Feelings about an interviewee may be aroused in an interviewer by the interviewee's resemblance to someone in the interviewer's past. This is an example of

(A) displacement
(B) projection
(C) illusion
(D) countertransference
(E) identification

16. The Minnesota multiphasic personality inventory (MMPI) is

(A) a subjective test
(B) a projective test
(C) an intelligence test
(D) a personality test
(E) a special aptitude test

17. Psychiatric rating scales that have been developed to evaluate symptoms and psychopathology include all the following EXCEPT

(A) Hamilton Rating Scale for Depression (Hamilton)
(B) Mental Status Examination Record (MSER)
(C) Present State Examination (PSE)
(D) Brief Psychiatric Rating Scale (BPRS)
(E) Social Adjustment Scale (SAS)

18. In documenting the mental status examination, all the following are reported except

(A) appearance
(B) behavior
(C) speech
(D) sleep pattern
(E) mood and affect

19. A person sitting alone and behaving as if listening intently suddenly begins to nod and mutter aloud. This person most likely is experiencing

(A) a delusion
(B) an illusion
(C) a hallucination
(D) an idea of reference
(E) a flight of ideas

20. In the assessment of the cognitive processes of a person suspected of having had an acute cerebral insult, it would be most important to

(A) test current verbal skills
(B) inquire about recent changes in mental function
(C) evaluate intelligence
(D) define the person's usual defenses and coping mechanisms
(E) search for long-term memory deficits

DIRECTIONS: Each question below contains four suggested responses of which **one or more** is correct. Select

A	if	**1, 2, and 3**	are correct
B	if	**1 and 3**	are correct
C	if	**2 and 4**	are correct
D	if	**4**	is correct
E	if	**1, 2, 3, and 4**	are correct

21. When there is a possible diagnosis of sleep apnea, it is particularly important to take a history from the spouse

(1) to determine whether the patient snores

(2) to evaluate the presence of marital discord

(3) to confirm the patient's daytime sleepiness

(4) to evaluate the spouse's typical sleep pattern

22. Psychological assessment can provide useful data in which of the following areas?

(1) Symptom severity and change

(2) Cognitive functioning

(3) Personality dynamics

(4) Psychiatric research

23. Diagnostic evaluation of a child with suspected mental retardation would include

(1) careful physical examination

(2) neurological examination

(3) examination of urine and blood for metabolic disorders

(4) psychological testing

24. A 40-year-old woman complains of fatigue, difficulty sleeping, and vague aches and pains and is preoccupied with her physical health. This clinical picture can suggest the presence of

(1) an occult carcinoma

(2) an endocrinopathy

(3) influenza

(4) depression

25. It is particularly important to evaluate thyroid function in patients presenting with

(1) compulsive rituals

(2) cognitive defects

(3) hysterical fits

(4) depression

26. Brain malfunctions may be indicated on the draw a person and Bender-Gestalt tests by the presence of

(1) perseveration

(2) difficulty in angulation

(3) oversimplification

(4) fragmentation

27. Assessment of psychiatric disorders according to the format detailed in the third edition of *Diagnostic and Statistical Manual of Mental Disorders (DSM III-R)* would include a statement or description of

(1) clinical diagnosis
(2) etiology
(3) best level of functioning in the last 12 months
(4) family history of mental illness

28. In psychiatry the electroencephalogram (EEG) has particular usefulness in the diagnosis of

(1) panic disorder
(2) delirium
(3) schizophrenia
(4) episodic disorders such as rage reactions

29. The differential diagnosis of violent homicidal behavior includes

(1) reserpine abuse
(2) amphetamine psychosis
(3) hypoglycemia
(4) catatonic excitement

30. Interpretation of responses to the Rorschach test may be used to help

(1) diagnose schizophrenia
(2) describe personality strengths
(3) reveal capacity for interpersonal relationships
(4) obtain an IQ measurement

31. In narcolepsy, the polysomnographic recording typically shows

(1) an absence of REM sleep
(2) anoxia
(3) spike and wave EEG recording
(4) an REM period shortly after sleep onset

DIRECTIONS: Each group of questions below consists of lettered headings followed by a set of numbered items. For each numbered item select the **one** lettered heading with which it is **most** closely associated. Each lettered heading may be used **once, more than once, or not at all.**

Questions 32–36

Match the following.

(A) Memory impairment
(B) Thought broadcasting
(C) Recurrent self-damaging acts
(D) Perfectionism
(E) Pathological jealousy

32. Paranoid personality disorder

33. Borderline personality disorder

34. Dementia

35. Schizophrenia

36. Obsessive compulsive personality disorder

Questions 37–40

Match the following.

(A) Prevalence
(B) Incidence
(C) Validity
(D) Primary prevention
(E) Secondary prevention

37. Early case finding and treatment to minimize duration of illness and to prevent permanent disability

38. The proportion of a population affected by a disorder at a given time

39. The proportion of a population that becomes affected by a disorder for the first time in a given period of time

40. Attempting to discover and eliminate the causes of mental illness

Questions 41–44

Match the following.

(A) Magical thinking
(B) Blocking
(C) Looseness of associations
(D) Derealization
(E) Depersonalization

41. Discontinuous and illogical stream of thoughts

42. A belief that thought alone can result in the accomplishment of certain wishes or activities

43. Sudden cessation of thinking in the middle of a discussion or sentence

44. The feeling that one is standing apart from oneself and observing one's own actions

DIRECTIONS: The group of questions below consists of four lettered headings followed by a set of numbered items. For each numbered item select

A	if the item is associated with	**(A) only**
B	if the item is associated with	**(B) only**
C	if the item is associated with	**both** (A) and (B)
D	if the item is associated with	**neither** (A) nor (B)

Each lettered heading may be used **once, more than once, or not at all.**

Questions 45–47

(A) Reliability
(B) Validity
(C) Both
(D) Neither

45. A measure of a test's ability to actually assess what it claims to

46. A measure of a test's reproducibility

47. A measure of the ability of a test's results to represent more than chance

Evaluation, Assessment, and Diagnosis

Answers

1. The answer is C. *(Michels, vol 1, chap 7, p 3.)* The most frequent reason for the use of psychological testing in a clinical psychiatric setting is assisting when there is uncertainty about diagnosis. Unlike semistructured interviews that generate broad clinical impressions, psychological testing yields specific, comparable information about diagnosis and severity of symptoms. It is not useful in determining medications or dosages or length of treatment. No diagnosis should be made strictly on the results of testing, but these results are useful when confronting difficult diagnostic problems.

2. The answer is D. *(Michels, vol 3, chap 51, pp 1–7.)* Brain-imaging techniques include x-ray, computed tomography (CT), emission tomography, nuclear magnetic resonance imaging (MRI), and positron emission tomography (PET). These techniques are widely employed in research studies of virtually all psychiatric conditions, but in most instances the findings do not have major diagnostic value. In the dementias, however, abnormalities on CT scan are present in a large number of patients, including those with dementias of the Alzheimer type. The findings are not specific enough to differentiate Alzheimer dementia from other senile dementias, or even at times from normal controls. The findings might be helpful in distinguishing dementia from the "pseudodementia" that may accompany severe depression.

3. The answer is C. *(Michels, vol 1, chap 7, p 9.)* Projective tests are standardized assessments using unstructured situations that allow for a patient's personality dynamics and style to emerge in a nonthreatening way. The Rorschach inkblot test is one of the best known; however, the thematic apperception test, draw a figure, and sentence completion test are also widely used and effective. The Zung is a test used for depression. It is a symptom-oriented self-assessment instrument that gathers data and is not projective in nature.

4. The answer is D. *(Kaplan, ed 4. p 127.)* Intelligence quotient (IQ) is a measure of a person's ability to function cognitively at the time of testing. Excessive fatigue, psychosis, and brain damage are three factors that can change a person's ability to function and thus affect IQ measurement. Neither environmental nor innate (genetic) origins of intelligence are measured directly by the IQ test. Skilled interpreters, however, can infer from the responses to an intelligence test how these and other factors, including poor motivation and poor rapport with an examiner, might have affected the IQ score.

5. The answer is D. *(Kaplan, ed 4. p 23.)* In the brain, the principal metabolite of norepinephrine is 3-methoxy-4-hydroxyphenylglycol (MHPG), which is excreted in the urine. Measuring urinary MHPG concentration can help in directing the pharmacological treatment of depressed persons. Depressed persons whose urinary MHPG levels are low are likely to respond to the antidepressant imipramine.

6. The answer is D. *(Kaplan, ed 4. p 575.)* In the United States, the rate of suicide in the general population is about 1 in 10,000 persons. Women attempt suicide nearly twice as often as men. Men, however, commit suicide three times as often as women.

7. The answer is A. *(Michels, vol 1, chap 68, p 1; vol 2, chap 87, p 1.)* A delusion is a false belief that is not supported by fact and cannot be challenged successfully by logic or reason. Delusions are not randomly selected but rather develop as a defense against or support for specific thoughts or experiences; consequently, delusional thinking is said to be under the control of emotional, not rational, forces. What might be viewed as delusional to members of one social or cultural group may not be viewed as such by members of a widely divergent culture or social system.

8. The answer is C. *(Michels, vol 1, chap 68, p 1.)* An illusion is a misinterpretation of an actual sensory stimulus. A person's emotional state and personality needs can play an important role in determining the presence and type of an illusion. For example, perhaps the girl described in the question thought she saw a bear in her room because the hospital is a frightening, hostile environment for her. Systemic disease states associated with confusion (certain types of poisoning, for instance) also can produce misperceptions of sensory images by interfering with proper functioning of the brain.

9. The answer is C. *(Kaplan, ed 4. pp 12, 13.)* Psychiatric illnesses in the families of identified patients are common. Recent twin and adoption studies have demonstrated the importance of genetic factors in psychiatric disorders. A family history of prior psychiatric contact can also provide insight into familial responses and attitudes toward treatment. The psychiatric disorders that are genetically transmitted, at least in part, include schizophrenia, affective disorders, alcoholism, and antisocial personality disorder. Lifetime risks of a given illness from immediate to more distant relatives of an affected person have been established. Such information provides the basis for genetic counselling.

10. The answer is D. *(Kaplan, ed 4. pp 575–580. Michels, vol 1, chap 71, pp 7, 8, 11.)* The phenomenon of suicide is shrouded in myth and misconception. For example, suicide is seldom attempted without prior warning. About 80 percent of persons who commit suicide clearly signal their intent, and 70 percent of depressed persons who commit suicide are in contact with a physician in the month before their death (nearly half in the preceding week). Suicidal behavior is not restricted to a particular personality type or psychiatric disorder. The tendency to commit suicide probably is not inherited, though suicide risk is higher than normal in members of a family with a history of suicide.

11. The answer is C. *(Michels, vol 2, chap 21, p 4.)* IQ scores are determined by taking the ratio of mental age to chronological age and multiplying by 100. This system of calculating the IQ was developed by W. L. Stern. The IQ is an indicator of relative brightness and can be used to compare children of different ages when mental age continues to increase in proportion to chronological age.

12. The answer is B. *(Kaplan, ed 4. pp 275–280. Michels, vol 3, chap 20, pp 5–6.)* Persons who have lost their spouses by death, divorce, or separation have suicide rates two to five times higher than married persons. The rate for single persons is twice that of those who are married. Suicide rates among married persons are lower in families with children than in those without. The suicide risk for widowed persons is greatest during the first year of bereavement.

13. The answer is A. *(Michels, vol 1, chap 32, pp 7–8.)* The woman described in the question likely is experiencing a hyperventilation syndrome. Hyperventilation, which commonly is associated with acute anxiety reactions, causes excessive loss of carbon dioxide and, as a result, leads to respiratory alkalosis. As blood pH rises ionization of calcium decreases, and clinical signs of tetany, such as painful muscle spasms in the hands, can become manifest. Other symptoms of hyperventilation include lightheadedness, headache, nausea, and tingling around the mouth and in the fingers and toes. Breathing into a paper bag reverses the symptoms because the reinspired air has a higher concentration of carbon dioxide than does normal air.

14. The answer is B. *(Michels, vol 3, chap 52, pp 8–10.)* Evaluation of a person's ability to engage in abstract thinking can be accomplished during a mental status examination by asking the person to compare two objects. Abstract responses group the objects in a common class (e.g., a table and a chair are both pieces of furniture.) Less abstract responses may describe the function of the items (a table and a chair both are used for eating), and concrete responses usually involve physical similarities between the items (a table and a chair both have legs). Although concrete responses in conjunction with other signs may be indicative of brain dysfunction or formal thought disorder, low educational level and low intelligence also are associated with concrete thinking. Psychotic persons occasionally respond with bizarre responses (a table and a chair both have millions of molecules).

15. The answer is D. *(Michels, vol 3, chap 36, pp 9–10.)* When feelings an interviewer develops for an interviewee are based on irrational, unconscious factors—for example, the interviewee's resemblance to someone in the interviewer's past—countertransference is said to be in operation. Sometimes these feelings can be positive; other times, negative. Although physicians and other psychotherapists are apt to like some patients more than others, inordinate feelings of anger or antagonism toward certain patients should prompt a search for what it is about the patients that is bothersome. The problems may relate more to an unresolved conflict within the interviewer than to the actual personality of the interviewee.

16. The answer is D. *(Michels, vol 1, chap 7, p 5; vol 1, chap 15, p 5.)* The Minnesota multiphasic personality inventory (MMPI) is a questionnaire designed to measure various dimensions of personality. Examination of the responses rates the test subject according to nine clinical scales. Because it has been administered to large numbers of normal and emotionally disturbed subjects, considerable normative data are available. It can be administered to a large group of persons at one time and scored by computer.

17. The answer is E. *(Kaplan, ed 4. pp 518, 522.)* Psychiatric rating scales have been developed to evaluate response to treatment in a variety of dimensions. They differ in a variety of ways, including their administration, content, and validity. The Social Adjustment Scale is oriented toward assessment of social contacts as opposed to specific psychiatric symptoms. The Hamilton Rating Scale for Depression was first published in 1960 and is the most widely used instrument by which interviewers rate and assess depression. The MSER is a computer-coded instrument that details the patient's symptomatology and current mental status. The BPRS, published by Overall and Gorham in 1962, is a commonly used research instrument that allows for the rating of a variety of dimensions of psychopathology.

18. The answer is D. *(Kaplan, ed 4. pp 118–120.)* The mental status examination has a standard format. Sleep pattern is important to assess in taking a psychiatric history, but it is not part of the written mental status examination. A cogent description of appearance, behavior, speech, mood, and affect is required.

19. The answer is C. *(Michels, vol 2, chap 87, p 1.)* A hallucination is the perception of a stimulus when, in fact, no sensory stimulus is present. Hallucinations can be auditory, visual, tactile, gustatory, olfactory, or kinesthetic. Auditory hallucinations are most commonly associated with psychotic illness, whereas visual, tactile, gustatory, and olfactory hallucinations are associated with neurologic disorders.

20. The answer is B. *(Kaplan, ed 4. pp 143, 144.)* Evaluation of a person suspected of having a neuropathological disorder should always include an assessment of cognitive function. Most useful diagnostically is a determination of how the person's cognitive ability has changed over time. For example, poor calculation skills in a person employed as an accountant may be more significant diagnostically than impaired arithmetic ability in a person with a long history of poor school performance. Thus, the assessment of *change* in cognitive function, rather than the specific cognitive function displayed on presentation, is crucial, because it enables clinicians to differentiate memory or other cognitive deficits of recent onset from those that are long-standing.

21. The answer is B (1, 3). *(Talbott, pp 746–747.)* In obstructive sleep apnea, one of the most common clinical findings is loud snoring. The patient may be unaware of this except from the description of others. These patients often thrash about in their sleep, gasp at the end of a period of apnea, and on occasion may wet the bed. The symptoms are very disruptive to the sleep of others, and thus an objective history may reveal information the patient is unable to provide.

22. The answer is E (all). *(Michels, vol 1, chap 7, p 1.)* Psychological assessment, which can be done with a wide variety of instruments, provides quantitative data in a variety of areas including symptom severity, cognitive functioning, and personality dynamics. Choosing the appropriate test is crucial and requires an understanding of the instrument and its limitations. Owing to the standardization of these tests, they are particularly useful in conducting psychiatric research.

23. The answer is E (all). *(Kaplan, ed 4. pp 709–721.)* A variety of conditions may simulate mental retardation. Careful diagnostic evaluation may reveal specific sensory handicaps, which may be mistaken for mental retardation. Chronic medical diseases can depress the child's functioning in several areas. Differential diagnostic expertise is required to rule out deafness or visual impairment in an infant or toddler. Speech deficits and cerebral palsy must be considered in a differential diagnosis. Any neurological disorder, including seizure disorders, may give an impression of mental retardation. The coexistence of severe behavioral manifestations of a childhood psychiatric disorder makes the evaluation very difficult.

24. The answer is E (all). *(Kaplan, ed 4. pp 248–251.)* The presence of vague aches and pains and preoccupation with somatic complaints can point to a diagnosis of depression. Often, depressed patients present clinically with a particular physical symptom, such as backache, and not with psychological disturbances. However, depressive syndromes also can be associated with medical conditions, such as occult malignancies, or be a manifestation of an endocrinopathy—particularly Cushing's syndrome, hypothyroidism, and hyperparathyroidism. Viral diseases, especially during their incubation and convalescent stages, also can produce a depressive syndrome. Thus, patients presenting with the signs and symptoms of depression should receive a thorough medical evaluation.

25. The answer is C (2, 4). *(Kaplan, ed 4. p 1170.)* Patients with hypothyroidism often experience a cognitive decline, which may be severe enough to present as a dementia. This condition is also strongly associated with depression that at times may be of psychotic proportions. The medical history, physical examination, and laboratory evaluation are extremely important in the evaluation of a patient who presents with symptoms of depression or cognitive decline. Hypothyroidism is not associated with compulsive rituals or with hysterical symptoms.

26. The answer is E (all). *(Kaplan, ed 4. pp 131, 132.)* Organic mental deficits may become apparent in the graphomotor productions of a person taking the draw a person or Bender-Gestalt tests. Figures may be conspicuously fragmented or oversimplified; difficulty in angulation, such as an inability to reproduce the angle between two figures, may appear. Affected persons may exhibit perseveration, which is the tendency to repeat the same design again and again, even if incorrect. Norms are available for the assessment of brain-damaged patients by the Bender-Gestalt test.

27. The answer is B (1, 3). *(American Psychiatric Association, ed 3-R. pp 15–24.)* *Diagnostic and Statistical Manual of Mental Disorders,* third edition *(DSM III-R),* attempts to categorize psychiatric disturbances according to a number of criteria. There is a separate "axis" to describe each of the following parameters: clinical diagnosis, personality diagnosis, associated medical conditions, severity of psychosocial stress, and best level of adaptive functioning currently and during the last year. This system is used to describe the clinical manifestations of a mental disorder and not how the disorder arose.

28. The answer is C (2, 4). *(Kaplan, ed 4. p 548.)* The EEG is a very useful diagnostic tool in distinguishing delirium from functional psychosis, and in the evaluation of episodic behavioral disorders. It may reveal organic pathology that is not demonstrable by other means, such as the CT scan. EEG abnormalities are not a usual finding in the neuroses or in schizophrenia.

29. The answer is C (2,4). *(Kaplan, ed 4. pp 190, 191. Michels, vol 1, chap 53, pp 12, 13, 15.)* Persons with catatonic schizophrenia are not always mute and stuporous. In the state of catatonic excitement, persons can become quite violent and destructive, toward themselves as well as others. Persons with amphetamine psychosis may be paranoid and violent. Mild hypoglycemia has a sedative effect, and severe hypoglycemia, though associated with signs of delirium and disorientation, quickly progresses to stupor. High-dose reserpine therapy (usually for hypertension) can lead to the development of depression, which is thought to be related to the depletion of brain stores of dopamine, serotonin, and norepinephrine. The depression usually remits when reserpine therapy is discontinued.

30. The answer is A (1, 2, 3). *(Michels, vol 1, chap 7, p 7; vol 2, chap 21, p 6.)* The test devised by the Swiss psychiatrist Hermann Rorschach consists of a set of ten inkblots that serve as stimuli for association. It is a projective test because subjects are forced to demonstrate how they think and perceive by finding meaningful symbols or shapes in a formless design. Responses can be compared with responses made by normal persons and persons with known disorders. Responses to cards that usually appear to present human forms may illuminate interpersonal attitudes or personality traits. Poor form perception and idiosyncratic or peculiar associations are examples of the type of responses made by schizophrenic persons. The Rorschach test is not a test of intelligence.

31. The answer is D (4). *(Talbott, pp 747–748.)* Patients with narcolepsy quite probably have a defect in REM inhibition. When sleep recordings are made, the patients typically show a sleep-onset REM period, or one that occurs very shortly after the onset of sleep. From 15 to 30 percent may also show some nocturnal myoclonus or sleep apnea.

32–36. The answers are: 32-E, 33-C, 34-A, 35-B, 36-D. *(American Psychiatric Association, ed 3-R. pp 103–107, 187–196, 337–338, 346–347, 354–356.)* The paranoid personality is characterized by litigiousness, expectation of harm, and guardedness. Because these patients question the loyalty of others, they may often experience pathological jealousy. During severe stress, transient psychotic symptoms may occur, but these do not persist.

The borderline personality as defined by *DSM-R* is characterized by emotional instability in a variety of areas including self-image. This results in unpredictable behavior that may be potentially self-damaging. Short-lived psychotic episodes have been described as micropsychotic. Delusional ideas that may occur are typically not bizarre.

Dementia typically interferes with social or occupational functioning because of significant memory impairment. Changes in personality and behavior may also occur. Reversibility of the memory impairment depends on the underlying cause. In most cases, however, short- and long-term memory deficits persist.

Schizophrenia is a major psychotic illness involving disturbance in psychological processes. There is a deterioration in level of functioning during some phases of the illness. Characteristic bizarre delusions such as thought broadcasting are more common in patients with schizophrenia than in patients with other psychotic disorders.

Finally, the compulsive personality is often described as perfectionistic. The patient may be preoccupied with rules, details, and orders. However, difficulty with decision making may manifest itself as part of the clinical presentation. The behavior of the compulsive personality reflects the need for organization and an urge for self-control. Such a patient has been called the orderly, controlling type, and this personality configuration is similar to the so-called type A personality.

37–40. The answers are: 37-E, 38-A, 39-B, 40-D. *(Nicholi, pp 762–767, 783.)* All the terms listed in the question group are particularly common to psychiatric epidemiology. Prevalence studies in psychiatry are far more common than incidence studies. Prevalence equals the cases in the population divided by the total population (cases plus noncases). It is generally measured at a given point in time (point prevalence) or over a given period of time (period prevalence). It counts both old and new cases, in contrast to incidence, which is a measure of the number of new cases that occur in a specified period.

Validity refers to the accuracy and verifiability of a study. It is usually demonstrated by agreement between two attempts to measure the same issue by different methods.

Primary prevention represents the attempt to discover and then eliminate the causes of illness, while secondary prevention relates to early case finding and treatment to shorten the illness and prevent permanent disability. Tertiary prevention is involved with rehabilitation.

41–44. The answers are: 41-C, 42-A, 43-B, 44-E. *(Kaplan, ed 4. pp 205, 207, 213.)* Looseness of associations refers to a string of thoughts that are disconnected in content and are illogical in their sequence. Circumstantiality is a disorder of association by which too little selective suppression of ideas allows too many associated concepts to come into consciousness. The connection between ideas, however, is usually logical and easy to follow.

Difficulty holding on to a train of thought—blocking—often manifests as an interruption in the middle of a thought. The sentence following such an interruption may have no relationship to what had just been said. Blocking, which is thought to be due to an intensification of anxiety, is not a conscious mechanism and thus not subject to conscious control.

Magical thinking is displayed by children, people affected by a variety of psychiatric conditions, and some primitive peoples. Essentially, it is a belief that specific thoughts, words, or gestures can directly lead to the fulfillment of wishes. Such thinking demonstrates an unrealistic understanding of the relationship between cause and effect.

Depersonalization is the sense of being outside of one's own body, observing oneself as an actor engaged in a role. This symptom may be manifested by people suffering from temporary anxiety, neurotic (especially phobic) people, and severely mentally ill people, such as certain schizophrenics. Some people with an organic brain disorder, such as temporal lobe epilepsy, may develop both depersonalization and derealization, the feeling that one's surroundings are unfamiliar or unreal.

45–47. The answers are: 45-B, 46-A, 47-D. *(Talbott, pp 72–74.)* When using assessment instruments, the clinician or researcher must be assured the test is valid and reliable. Validity refers to the test's ability to assess what it claims to be assessing. Reliability refers to the reproducibility of results at various times. An unreliable test will not produce consistent results. Statistical significance refers to the results and how often they would happen by chance. A p value of less than 0.05 is statistically significant and means the results would only happen 5 times out of 100 by chance.

Human Behavior: Theories of Personality and Development

DIRECTIONS: Each question below contains five suggested responses. Select the **one best** response to each question.

48. The large majority of mentally retarded persons are mildly retarded, with IQs on standard psychological tests of

(A) below 20
(B) 20 to 34
(C) 35 to 49
(D) 50 to 70
(E) 71 to 85

49. Tourette's disorder is characterized by

(A) onset between ages 15 and 30
(B) sleep disturbance
(C) sexual dysfunction
(D) multiple motor and vocal tics
(E) episodes of panic

50. Which of the following theorists primarily focused on the maturation of the sense of self from infantile fragility and fragmentation into the cohesive and stable structure of adulthood?

(A) Piaget
(B) Erikson
(C) Freud
(D) Klein
(E) Kohut

51. According to modern psychoanalytic theory, narcissism in children is

(A) a syndrome characterized by excessive masturbation
(B) a part of the development of all children
(C) first manifested during the phallic phase
(D) unusual except in psychotic children
(E) a pathological trait usually due to overinvolved maternal care

52. The early studies of Réné Spitz suggested that

(A) disturbed mothers are instrumental in causing behavioral problems in early infancy
(B) infants reared with little maternal contact are more susceptible to infections and behavioral problems
(C) infants reared in an institutional setting are likely to become autistic
(D) the number of toys available to infants is a crucial factor in their development
(E) environmental variables have little impact on the health of infants

53. All the following statements concerning children's IQ scores are true EXCEPT that

(A) the scores can vary widely if an individual child is tested more than once
(B) the scores can increase over time in children who are highly motivated
(C) the scores correlate fairly well with achievement in school
(D) the scores are determined predominantly by heredity
(E) the mean of the scores remains fairly constant within a given group

54. Children diagnosed as having attention deficit disorder, also called minimal brain dysfunction (MBD), would be LEAST likely to display which of the following signs?

(A) Impulsivity
(B) Hyperactivity
(C) Emotional lability
(D) Severe neurological deficits
(E) Perceptual motor impairments

DIRECTIONS: Each question below contains four suggested responses of which **one or more** is correct. Select

A	if	**1, 2, and 3**	are correct
B	if	**1 and 3**	are correct
C	if	**2 and 4**	are correct
D	if	**4**	is correct
E	if	**1, 2, 3, and 4**	are correct

55. True statements about REM sleep include which of the following?

(1) The proportion and duration of REM sleep decrease from birth to adulthood

(2) Most adults spend 80 to 100 minutes each night in REM sleep, which is associated with three to six separate dreams

(3) REM sleep is not the only state in which dreams can occur

(4) Depressed patients who are deprived of REM sleep have a marked worsening of their condition

56. Patients with Down's syndrome often display

(1) chromosomal abnormalities

(2) hypotonia and hyperflexibility

(3) a flat nasal bridge

(4) shortness of ear length

57. True statements about the human immune system include

(1) exposure to psychosocial stress can alter a variety of components of immune function

(2) it is highly unlikely that early life experiences will alter the immune system in later life

(3) immune response has been found to be subject to conditioning effects

(4) immune abnormalities have been shown to be involved in the pathogenesis of schizophrenia

58. True statements about sleepwalking include

(1) 15 percent of children from the ages of 5 to 12 sleepwalk at least once

(2) sleepwalking in children is usually not associated with psychopathology

(3) sleepwalking is potentially dangerous and requires precautions to protect the child

(4) a psychological cause is suggested when sleepwalking begins in adolescence or adulthood

59. Children with attention-deficit disorder

(1) often fidget and are restless
(2) persevere in a single activity
(3) often talk excessively
(4) are obsessively careful to avoid dangerous play

60. In psychoanalytic theory, the superego

(1) contains the ego ideal, an internalized set of standards
(2) contains the unconscious conscience
(3) demands punishment in the form of guilt and shame
(4) is the source of the psychological defense mechanisms that repress unacceptable impulses

61. True statements about the expressive movements of the human face in infancy include

(1) smiling and expressions of disgust appear at birth
(2) by 9 months of age infants can produce most adult emotional expressions
(3) babies who are blind at birth display expressions of anger, fear, sadness, and happiness
(4) by the age of 2 months, infants are using facial expression to communicate with adults

62. True statements regarding the differences between men and women include which of the following?

(1) Women have a higher prevalence rate of affective disorders
(2) Men have a higher prevalence rate of anxiety disorders
(3) Prevalence rates of personality disorders are consistently higher for men
(4) Women have a prevalence rate of schizophrenia that is twice that for men

63. The structural theory of the psyche, introduced by Freud in 1923, is characterized by which of the following statements?

(1) It focuses on the concepts of libidinal energy and cathexis
(2) It hypothesizes that the mind is composed of three entities: id, ego, and superego
(3) It identifies the existence of oral, anal, and phallic phases of psychosexual development
(4) Its introduction added emphasis to the importance of the ego in mental functioning

64. Current family theory views the family as a structured system whose functions include

(1) emancipational functions
(2) communicative functions
(3) nurturant functions
(4) recuperative functions

SUMMARY OF DIRECTIONS

A	B	C	D	E
1,2,3	1,3	2,4	4	All are
only	only	only	only	correct

65. Psychoanalytic theory describes the ego as a coherent system of functions, including

(1) regulation of instinctual drives
(2) defense formation
(3) formation of relationships
(4) adaptation to reality

66. Homosexuality is a controversial subject within the psychiatric profession. Which of the following general statements can be said to conform to the predominant psychiatric understanding of homosexual persons?

(1) They suffer from a serious mental disorder
(2) There is a well-established biological and hormonal etiology
(3) They are more likely to seduce children than are heterosexuals
(4) Their overall level of psychopathology is not significantly greater than that of heterosexuals

67. Freud's theory of infantile sexual development can be described by which of the following statements?

(1) It postulates that sexuality begins in early infancy
(2) It links neurosis with disturbance in psychosexual development
(3) It describes the earliest sexuality as centered in the mouth, lips, and tongue
(4) It suggests that masturbation normally begins during the latency period

68. Childhood stuttering is accurately described by which of the following statements?

(1) Affected children usually have obsessive compulsive personality traits
(2) Affected children often outgrow the problem
(3) Girls are affected more commonly than boys
(4) A family history of stuttering frequently is elicited

69. According to classic psychoanalytic theory, correct statements about the phallic phase of development include which of the following?

(1) It marks the start of the oedipal conflict
(2) It occurs after 5 years of age
(3) It is characterized by sexual curiosity and comparison
(4) It does not occur in girls

70. The analytic psychology of Carl Jung explores in depth which of the following concepts?

(1) Archetypal modes of experience
(2) Introversion-extroversion
(3) The "shadow"
(4) Character armor

71. Primary process thinking is a psychoanalytic concept describing mental activity that is

(1) typically unconscious
(2) prelogical and primitive
(3) manifested in dreams
(4) prominent in psychosis

72. Current evidence suggests that genetic (inherited) factors may play an important role in which of the following disorders?

(1) Bipolar disorder
(2) Tourette's syndrome
(3) Schizophrenia
(4) Alzheimer's disease

73. The psychological development of adolescents is far from a uniform process. Normal psychological growth patterns for adolescent males include which of the following?

(1) Intermittent surges of psychological growth
(2) Continuous and steady psychological growth
(3) Tumultuous psychological growth
(4) Episodic identity diffusion

74. Harry Stack Sullivan's theory of personality development is characterized by which of the following concepts?

(1) An emphasis on the importance of interpersonal relations
(2) A conviction that the basic structure of personality is fixed by about 5 years of age
(3) A concern with the developmental impact of social position and lifestyle
(4) A focus on ego psychology

75. The developmental theories of Erikson and Freud differ in that

(1) Erikson minimizes the role of the unconscious, while Freud emphasizes it
(2) Erikson emphasizes the interplay of cultural factors with individual psychological development to a greater degree than Freud
(3) Erikson's is a behavioral theory, while Freud's is an analytic theory
(4) Erikson places greater emphasis than Freud on ego structures

76. Correct statements concerning infantile autism include which of the following?

(1) It may occur during the first few months of life
(2) It usually is not associated with language disturbances
(3) It may manifest itself in resistance to minor environmental changes
(4) Affected infants form abnormally intense attachments to adults

SUMMARY OF DIRECTIONS

A	B	C	D	E
1,2,3 only	1,3 only	2,4 only	4 only	All are correct

77. Correct statements about adopted children include which of the following?

(1) They should be told of their adoption at an early age, according to most experts
(2) They usually search for their biological parents only if their adoptive family relations are seriously troubled
(3) They are more likely to display behavioral problems, learning difficulties, and minimal brain dysfunction than are nonadopted children
(4) They often are painfully disillusioned if they succeed in finding and meeting their biological parents

78. Battered or abused children are

(1) abused most commonly by their fathers
(2) usually from very poor families
(3) most frequently between 3 and 6 years of age when the diagnosis is made
(4) typically born to parents who were abused when they were children

79. Correct statements concerning the latency stage of development include which of the following?

(1) It follows resolution of the Oedipus complex
(2) It consolidates identification with the parent of the same sex
(3) It involves wider peer contact
(4) It is the phase of identity crisis

80. In psychoanalytic theory, the anal phase of development, which occurs between the ages of approximately 1 and 3 years, is characterized by

(1) struggles over routines
(2) depressive episodes
(3) striving for independence
(4) head banging

DIRECTIONS: Each group of questions below consists of lettered headings followed by a set of numbered items. For each numbered item select the **one** lettered heading with which it is **most** closely associated. Each lettered heading may be used **once, more than once, or not at all.**

Questions 81–83

The concept of defenses is central to psychoanalytic theory. Match each of the definitions below to the defense mechanism being described.

(A) Acting out
(B) Rationalization
(C) Isolation
(D) Repression
(E) Sublimation

81. The unconscious exclusion of an idea or feeling from conscious awareness

82. The intrapsychic separation of affect and mental content

83. The direct behavioral expression of an unconscious impulse

Questions 84–87

Match the following.

(A) John Bowlby
(B) Jean Piaget
(C) Anna Freud
(D) Margaret Mahler
(E) Arnold Gesell

84. Separation-individuation theory of early development

85. Cognitive development

86. Defense mechanisms

87. Normative developmental theory

Questions 88–91

Match the following.

(A) Core-gender identity
(B) Gender-role behavior
(C) Gender-role identity
(D) Sexual identity
(E) Sex print

88. The internal experience of sexual arousal patterns and self-labeling

89. The inner conviction that one is a male or one is a female

90. The individual's self-evaluation of psychological maleness or femaleness

91. The objective patterns of sexuality

Questions 92–95

For each age below, select the psychosocial crisis, as described by Erikson, with which it is most likely to be associated.

(A) Identity versus role confusion
(B) Generativity versus stagnation
(C) Integrity versus despair
(D) Initiative versus guilt
(E) Industry versus inferiority

92. 5 years of age

93. 15 years of age

94. 40 years of age

95. 65 years of age

Questions 96–99

Match the following.

(A) Neutralization
(B) Wish fulfillment
(C) Identification
(D) Secondary gain
(E) Overdetermination

96. The concept that a symptom may have a number of different origins and meanings

97. The process by which libidinal and aggressive drives are mastered and provide conflict-free energy

98. The benefit derived as a result of neurotic illness

99. The unconscious process by which persons pattern themselves after others

Human Behavior: Theories of Personality and Development

Answers

48. The answer is D. *(American Psychiatric Association, ed 3-R. pp 28–33.)* Mild retardation refers to the condition of those persons whose IQ tests are between 50 and 70 on standard tests such as the Stanford-Binet or Wechsler. These people constitute about 85 percent of those with mental retardation and are often not distinguishable from other children until later in childhood. They can be expected to learn academic skills up to approximately the sixth-grade level, and with proper social and vocational education they can achieve minimum levels of self-support as adults.

49. The answer is D. *(American Psychiatric Association, ed 3-R. pp 79–80.)* Tourette's disorder has its onset before age 21 and is characterized by multiple motor and vocal tics that have been present during the illness, although not necessarily concurrently. A tic is defined as an involuntary, sudden, rapid, recurrent, non-rhythmic, and stereotyped motor movement or vocalization. It is experienced as irresistible and exacerbated by stress. Sometimes it can be suppressed. Tics are usually diminished during sleep.

50. The answer is E. *(Kaplan, ed 4. pp 178–183. Michels, vol 1, chap 1, pp 2–15.)* Heinz Kohut developed a variant of psychoanalysis that has had a powerful influence on modern psychoanalytic treatment. He believed that psychic development was primarily organized around the developmental vicissitudes of the self, primarily in the relationship to interactions with self-objects. The most important self-object of infancy is the mother. Freudian psychoanalysis postulated a sequence of psychosexual development that stressed unconscious conflict and the influence of sexual and aggressive drives. Erik Erikson elaborated the role of culture in shaping the meaning of these drives throughout the life cycle. Melanie Klein is associated with the object-relations school of psychoanalysis, especially a minute dissection of the early relationship of the child and mother. Piaget is particularly known for his work on the development of intellect.

51. The answer is B. *(Kaplan, ed 4. pp 374–377.)* The concept of narcissism, or self-love, is a major one in modern psychoanalytic theory. Narcissism, viewed as a normal part of the development of all children, beginning in infancy, need not be pathological. Although linked to autoeroticism, narcissism does not imply genital sexuality.

52. The answer is B. *(Nicholi, p 609.)* Réné A. Spitz's pioneering studies on the effects of institutionalization on infants compared three groups of children: those reared by their delinquent mothers in the nursery of a penal institution; those reared in a foundling home with no maternal contact; and those reared in two-parent home environments. The infants raised in the foundling home showed a markedly higher incidence of disease and developmental delay. The key factor that differentiated this group from the others was the lack of maternal contact and not the type of mothering, institutional setting, or play environment.

53. The answer is D. *(Kaplan, ed 4. p 505.)* IQ scores, which correlate fairly well with school achievement, can vary widely in an individual child tested more than once. In one study, the scores of more than two-thirds of the tested children varied by more than 15 points over a specified period of time. Despite such individual variation, however, the mean IQ of a given group remains quite constant. Children who at 5 years of age display high levels of independence and self-initiative are more likely to show subsequent IQ gains. There have not been any adequate studies demonstrating that IQ is determined predominantly by heredity.

54. The answer is D. *(Kaplan, ed 4. pp 1684–1690.)* Attention deficit disorder is characterized by hyperactivity, distractibility, emotional lability, perceptual motor defects, learning problems, and short attention span. Neurological examination of affected children may reveal no abnormalities or may show minimal, nonspecific signs, including hearing and speech deficits and coordination problems. Electroencephalography often reveals a variety of nonspecific abnormalities, though testing in a significant percentage of affected children provides normal results.

55. The answer is A (1, 2, 3). *(Michels, vol 3, chap 60, pp 2–10.)* Sleep is usually classified into rapid and nonrapid eye movement (REM and NREM) sleep. Most adults have three to six dreams per night during an average of 1 to 2 hours of REM sleep. Dreaming is particularly associated with REM sleep, but it can also occur during NREM sleep, when it has a tendency to be more conceptual than perceptual. The normal newborn's REM sleep is about 50 percent of total sleep, but by 2 to 3 years of age the child reaches the adult level of 20 to 25 percent. Depriving depressed patients of REM sleep appears to have an antidepressant effect.

56. The answer is E (all). *(Kaplan, ed 4. p 1645.)* The diagnosis of Down's syndrome is ultimately made by study of the chromosomes. While there is no physical anomaly invariably present, the vast majority of patients display hypotonia, hyperflexibility, midface depression, and short ear length. Other common physical findings include oblique palpebral fissures, loose skin on the back of the neck, and gaps between the first and second toes.

57. The answer is B (1, 3). *(Michels, vol 2, chap 128, pp 1–14.)* The effects of stress on the immune system, as well as responsiveness to conditioning, are well established in animals. Evidence is similarly accumulating regarding humans. A number of investigators have demonstrated that early life experience may alter the immune system so that the effects persist into later life. Research has failed to yet establish a relationship between pathology in the immune system and schizophrenia. However, it is clear that the immune system is modulated by psychosocial events via effects on the central nervous system and endocrine processes.

58. The answer is E (all). *(Michels, vol 2, chap 43, pp 6–7; vol 2, chap 52, p 6.)* While 15 percent of children will sleepwalk at least once, in only a much smaller percentage does it become recurrent and persistent. Usually the problem will resolve spontaneously by the age of 15, though sometimes it becomes associated with the problem of night terrors. Studies of adult somnambulists have found a large percentage with demonstrable psychiatric problems. It is quite possible for a child to be injured while sleepwalking, since it is not purposeful behavior. It has been postulated that sleepwalking and night terrors share a common physiologic origin for which there may be a genetic predisposition.

59. The answer is B (1, 3). *(American Psychiatric Association, ed 3-R. pp 50–53.)* Attention-deficit disorder has its onset before age 7 and is a disturbance of at least 6 months' duration. The symptoms include hyperactivity, impulsive speech and behavior, and easy distractibility. Patients often have difficulty in maintaining attention on one activity and in listening to others. An important management problem relates to the tendency to engage in dangerous behavior without considering the consequences.

60. The answer is A (1, 2, 3). *(Michels, vol 1, chap 1, p 9.)* The superego is the "site" of the ego ideal and of the conscience. It sits in judgment as to whether one's behavior and wishes are right, wrong, good, bad, or shameful. It is a largely unconscious process and does not distinguish between thoughts and acts. For this reason, it produces guilt about wish and fantasy, not merely about the person's deeds.

61. The answer is E (all). *(Kaplan, ed 4. p 243.)* There is an extensive literature on the facial expressions of infants, and the preponderance of evidence suggests that this activity is innate. Even blind babies will smile while fixating toward their mother's voice, in addition to showing other emotional expressiveness. While visual learning provides an important element in the development of normal expressive behavior, innate factors are clearly operative.

62. The answer is B (1, 3). *(Kaplan, ed 4. p 270.)* The differences between males and females as to prevalence of mental and emotional disorders reflect a complex interaction between biological and sociocultural factors. The sexes are treated differently with respect to expectations, social roles, social opportunities, and so forth. All these factors operate throughout the life cycle to shape behavior and responses to the environment. Women have been shown to have a greater prevalence rate of affective disorders and anxiety disorders, and a lesser rate of personality disorders. There are slight and perhaps not significantly different rates for schizophrenia and organic brain syndromes associated with aging.

63. The answer is C (2, 4). *(Kaplan, ed 4. pp 1336–1337.)* In 1923, Freud presented the theory that the psyche is composed of three basic structures: id, ego, and superego. The structural theory states that instinctual drives arise in the id, which is concerned with the pursuit of gratification. The ego was conceived as an entity of executive function, regulating drives and maintaining relations with the external world. The superego maintains parental values and prohibitions. With the presentation of the structural model, Freud abandoned his topographic theory, a simpler model that focused on the conscious and unconscious regions of the mind. The new theory represented an increasing emphasis on the importance of the ego in mental functioning. Freud's concepts of libidinal energy, cathexis, and the phases of psychosexual development preceded the structural theory.

64. The answer is E (all). *(Kaplan, ed 4. pp 279–287.)* Family functions include marital, nurturant, relational, communicative, emancipational, and recuperative functions. A successful marriage satisfies the needs of both partners, so that they can jointly address family tasks. The physical, emotional, intellectual, and psychological nurturance of children is a critical family task. Teaching children the basics of communication is a central educative family task, as is facilitating the gradual emancipation of children. The family also must provide opportunities for shared relaxation, informal and creative interchange, and recuperation from the stresses of work.

65. The answer is E (all). *(Kaplan, ed 4. pp 387–391.)* The ego mediates between a person's instincts and the outside world. It is the part of the personality that perceives stimuli and can respond to them through control of both the id and voluntary muscular responses. Its many functions include reality testing, the formation and regulation of defenses, and the establishment of relationships with others.

66. The answer is D(4). *(Kaplan, ed 4. pp 1058–1063.)* The current view of the American Psychiatric Association is that homosexuality should not be considered a mental disorder unless it causes the homosexual person persistent distress. The rate of homosexual pedophilia (seduction of children) is no higher than the rate of heterosexual pedophilia. Similarly, rates and types of psychopathology appear to be no different in homosexuals than in heterosexuals. The roots of homosexual behavior are obscure and a matter of considerable controversy.

67. The answer is A (1, 2, 3). *(Kaplan, ed 4. pp 358–362.)* Freud postulated the existence of three phases of infantile psychosexual development. The oral phase lasts for the first year to year and a half of life, a time during which an infant's needs, perceptions, and pleasures are centered in the mouth, lips, and tongue. Masturbation begins in early infancy and peaks in the phallic phase and again at puberty. Psychoanalytic theory links neurosis with disturbances in psychosexual development— Freud observed that many of his patients had distorted memories of early sexual experiences, confusing infantile sexual fantasy with actual events.

68. The answer is C (2, 4). *(Kaplan, ed 4. pp 1716–1719.)* The causes of stuttering are not known. Although the incidence of stuttering in the relatives of stutterers is higher than in the general population, the genetic contribution to the development of stuttering is unclear. Stuttering affects boys more often and more chronically than girls. Treatment is controversial; however, 40 percent or more of affected young children eventually outgrow the difficulty. No particular personality classification is typical of persons who stutter.

69. The answer is B (1, 3). *(Kaplan, ed 4. p 361.)* According to classic psychoanalytic theory, the phallic phase of development begins at approximately 3 years of age and lasts about 2 years. During this time the erotic preoccupations of both boys and girls shift from the anal to the genital areas of the body. Children in this phase become sexually curious, comparing themselves with each other and with their parents. They compete for the attention of the parent of the opposite sex and are buffeted by intense and conflict-laden relations with both parents. This phenomenon, the Oedipus complex, plays a critical role in the pathogenesis of neurotic disorders.

70. The answer is A (1, 2, 3). *(Kaplan, ed 4. pp 433–440, 455.)* The analytic psychology of Carl Jung, who was a contemporary and an associate of Freud, explores the idea of archetypal modes of experience as embodied in universal symbols, myths, religious ideas, and other forms of expression. He also suggested that introversion and extroversion are complementary forces present in varying proportions in each person. Another of Jung's concepts is that of the "shadow," which symbolizes some of the rejected, unacceptable, and perhaps unconscious aspects of the psyche. The analysis of character armor is a central aspect of the work of Wilhelm Reich.

71. The answer is E (all). *(Kaplan, ed 4. pp 354–355, 1334, 1433.)* Psychoanalytic theory describes primary process thinking as mental activity related to the id. It is prelogical, timeless, primitive, and associated with the tendency to seek immediate gratification. It is characteristic of infancy, dreams, and psychotic thinking, but it is largely unconscious in normal waking life. Secondary process thinking is related to the activity of the ego. It is organized, logical, responsive to the demands of reality, and, unlike primary process thinking, usually conscious.

72. The answer is E (all). *(Kaplan, ed 4. pp 36–41.)* Although conclusive proof is lacking, studies of twins, adopted children, and biochemical data suggest that many psychiatric disorders have a significant genetic component. The data are particularly strong for affective disorders. Current evidence indicates there are at least three genetic forms of bipolar disorder. Data from family histories and from biochemical studies suggest that Tourette's syndrome has an inherited basis. Schizophrenia remains more controversial, but a reasonable interpretation of the evidence indicates that both inherited *and* environmental factors contribute to the disorder. Although a clear-cut pattern of genetic predisposition to Alzheimer's disease has not emerged, well-documented familial cases exist, some of which follow an autosomal dominant pattern of inheritance.

73. The answer is A (1, 2, 3). *(Kaplan, ed 4. pp 1608–1613, 1762–1764.)* Longitudinal studies of middle-class adolescent boys have suggested three normative psychological growth patterns. The boys associated with the continuous-growth pattern passed smoothly and steadily through adolescence. The surgent-growth group was characterized by developmental spurts punctuated by periods of regression. These boys had higher levels of conflict and distress than had the boys in the continuous-growth group. The tumultuous-growth group showed a marked tendency to undergo emotional upheavals, engage in family conflicts, and be distrustful of others. All three of these patterns are considered to be within the normal range. Significant identity diffusion represents a potentially serious disruption of development and is considered to be psychopathological.

74. The answer is B (1, 3). *(Kaplan, ed 4. pp 426–432.)* Harry Stack Sullivan is best known for his theory of personality development, which emphasizes the central importance of interpersonal relations. Sullivan believed that the first 5 years of life, though crucial to psychological development, do not fully fix personality; instead, personality continues to develop and change throughout adolescence and even into adulthood. He emphasized the influence of social position and conditions on development. Sullivan's theory focuses on a complex concept of the self, which differs in important respects from the psychoanalytic concept of the ego.

75. The answer is C (2, 4). *(Colarusso, pp 27–33. Kaplan, ed 4. pp 371–374.)* The developmental theories of both Freud and Erikson are psychoanalytic and acknowledge the role of the unconscious. Erikson, however, is more concerned with the individual's development as it relates to the surrounding cultural milieu. Consistent with more recent psychoanalytic theory, Erikson also emphasizes ego psychology in his formulations.

76. The answer is B (1, 3). *(Kaplan, ed 4. pp 1673–1679.)* Infantile autism manifests itself quite early in life and is often associated with a language disturbance. Children with infantile autism have an extreme desire to avoid all change. These children tend to lack any interest in forming normal attachments to other people.

77. The answer is B (1, 3). *(Kaplan, ed 4. pp 1829–1831.)* The consensus among adoption experts is that adopted children should be told of their adoption sometime between 2 and 4 years of age. Adopted children appear to develop behavioral problems and learning difficulties more often than other children. Moreover, adopted children born to teenage mothers may have an increased incidence of a variety of neurological disorders, perhaps because of poor prenatal and obstetrical care. Mature adoptees usually are interested in their biological parents (birth parents) and may search for them. Most adoptees find reunion with their birth parents a positive experience that often leads them to form a closer relationship with their adoptive parents.

78. The answer is D (4). *(Kaplan, ed 4. pp 1816–1823.)* Although child abuse can affect children of any age, children less than 3 years of age are affected most frequently and most severely. Mothers, more often than fathers, are the abusers. Abusing parents commonly were abused when they were children, and families in which child abuse occurs can be found in all socioeconomic strata.

79. The answer is A (1, 2, 3). *(Kaplan, ed 4. p 361.)* The latency stage of development follows the resolution of the Oedipus complex and lasts until adolescence (i.e., from approximately 5 to 13 years of age). During this period, children consolidate their sense of identification with parents of the same sex and develop an active fantasy life. Cognitive skills are expanded, and contacts with significant, extrafamilial figures (e.g., in school) widen. Identity crisis is a term coined by Erikson to describe another stage of development—adolescence.

80. The answer is B (1, 3). *(Kaplan, ed 4. p 360.)* In the anal phase of development, children struggle with their parents over eating, toilet training, sleeping, and other situations in which their autonomy is brought into question. Whether depressive-type episodes occur during the anal period is controversial; the clinicians who believe that these episodes do occur consider their presence highly pathological. Because head banging occurs more frequently earlier in life, its occurrence during the anal phase should suggest the need for psychiatric evaluation.

81–83. The answers are: 81-D, 82-C, 83-A. *(Kaplan, ed 4. pp 388–390.)* Psychoanalytic theory postulates that every person, normal or neurotic, uses defenses. Some defenses, such as altruism (vicarious gratification by service to others) and sublimation (gratification of a potentially objectionable impulse by socially acceptable means), are considered to be mature and healthy. Repression, isolation, and rationalization are neurotic defenses. Repression, which plays a primary role in the pathogenesis of hysteria, involves the unconscious exclusion of a thought or feeling from conscious awareness. It often is associated with symbolic behavior representing expression of the repressed mental content. Isolation involves separating painful feelings from the thoughts provoking them. Both the thoughts and attendant affect may be excluded from awareness or the affect may be displaced onto a different thought altogether. Rationalization involves supporting unacceptable ideas or behavior by basically inaccurate but plausible explanations. Acting out is an immature defense in which an inner conflict can be partially and transiently relieved by unconscious expression in impulsive action.

84–87. The answers are: 84-D, 85-B, 86-C, 87-E. *(Talbott, pp 94–102.)* Margaret Mahler developed her separation-individuation theory to describe the process whereby the infant differentiates from being enmeshed psychologically with the mother to a condition of separateness and relative independence. Bowlby was interested in the reactive effects that ensued when children were separated from their mother or her surrogate, as well as the nature of the maternal tie. Piaget was an early investigator who developed a very comprehensive theory of the stages of cognitive development. Anna Freud made an important contribution to psychoanalysis by her study of children, and by delineating the ego's mechanisms of defense. She was interested in how the child organizes behavior in an affective climate and in relation to others. This helped to develop the foundations of object-relations theory in psychoanalysis. This theory focuses on the developmental vicissitudes of the child's developmental mental representations of significant adults (objects) such as parents. Gesell observed child development in a cross-sectional fashion, describing a normative timetable as to what children can do at varying ages. He divided behavior into motor, personal-social, adaptive, and language functions.

88–91. The answers are: 88-D, 89-A, 90-C, 91-E. *(Michels, vol 1, chap 46, pp 1–2.)* Sexual identity refers to how a person subjectively experiences his or her sexual arousal patterns. It includes an awareness of what is experienced as erotic and desirable and is a part of one's overall sense of self. For example, a person who experiences both homosexual and heterosexual erotic arousal might consult a psychiatrist because of confusion about sexual identity.

Core-gender identity reflects a self-image of one's biological sex. It therefore represents the person's self-designation as being female or male. Generally it corresponds to biological sex, but it may be ambiguous in certain hermaphroditic conditions as well as in gender identity disorders such as transsexualism.

Gender-role identity refers to a person's self-image and self-evaluation that results in a belief that "I am male" or "I am female." It develops well into adulthood and fluctuates sometimes as a reflection of the person's evaluation of feelings, behavior, and performance. It is closely connected to the degree to which one feels one has adequately met the prescribed cultural role.

The sex print refers to objective patterns of sexuality. It is more comprehensive than preference for a particular sexual object or a specific sexual activity, but is the deep-rooted script that is most able to elicit erotic desire. It contributes to the person's sexual identity (subjective self-labeling), but forms the objective patterns that determine the substance of the person's sexual fantasies and behavior.

92–95. The answers are: 92-D, 93-A, 94-B, 95-C. *(Colarusso, pp 27–33. Kaplan, ed 4. pp 371–374.)* Erikson described the personality development of humans in terms of eight major, sequential stages. While acknowledging Freud's psychosexual developmental theory, Erikson broadened the scope of his formulations by including social factors outside the parent-child triad, by shifting the emphasis from psychopathological constructs to issues of normal growth and development, and by concluding that the process of development is a lifelong one. The resolution of each of the eight stages of development depends, Erikson said, on mastery of prior stages and influences the course of subsequent stages.

In the oral-sensory stage (the first year of life), trust versus mistrust is the important issue. In the second stage, corresponding to the Freudian anal period, successful resolution results in autonomy; problems in this stage can result in shame or self-doubt. The third stage lasts through the fifth year of life and parallels the Freudian period characterized by the emergence of the Oedipus complex. Erikson describes the task of this stage as the healthy growth of initiative. During latency, years 6 to 11, industry versus inferiority is the important psychosocial crisis. Building on the autonomy and initiative of earlier stages, children approach the tasks of adult life. Whether industry flourishes or feelings of inferiority arise depends on children's interactions with teachers and peers, as well as with parents. Erikson's ideas about the development of identity during adolescence are particularly well known. He felt that, during this period, adolescents try to integrate and clarify their own identities in relation to their parents, peers, and members of the opposite sex; if they are unsuccessful, role confusion can result.

Although Freud believed that the reworking of the Oedipus complex in adolescence was the final stage of development, Erikson saw development continuing into adulthood. He saw intimacy versus isolation to be the primary crisis of young adults. During the years of middle age, generativity versus stagnation is the key issue. Erikson emphasized the importance not only of rearing children but also of engaging in activities to help others, particularly new generations. In the final stage, people reflect on their lives. Adequate resolution of the stages of intimacy and generativity provides contentment in this stage (integrity); poor resolution can foster despair and a debilitating fear of death.

96–99. The answers are: 96-E, 97-A, 98-D, 99-C. *(Kaplan, ed 4. pp 351–354, 390, 498, 920.)* Each of the terms listed in the question describes a concept important to psychoanalytic theory. Neutralization is the term suggested by Heinz Hartmann to describe the process by which libidinal and aggressive drives are mastered, thus freeing energy for the ego. This concept is important in helping to explain nondefensive ego functioning. Overdetermination describes the concept that mental phenomena, such as neurotic symptoms and dreams, have multiple causes and thus have multiple meanings.

Identification is a defense that plays an important role in normal development. It involves unconscious patterning after another person, producing structural change in the ego.

Primary gain refers to the relief of tension and conflict produced by the development of neurotic symptoms. In addition to the internal reduction of distress, neurotic persons may attempt to derive compensation or gratification from the external world (secondary gain) as a result of their suffering. Examples of secondary gain include an increase in attention and sympathy, relief from burdensome obligations, and monetary compensation.

Wish fulfillment is the term used by Freud to describe the primary goal of dreams.

Human Behavior: Biological and Related Sciences

DIRECTIONS: Each question below contains five suggested responses. Select the **one best** response to each question.

100. Synaptic communication in the brain is accomplished via which of the following mechanisms?

(A) Chemical only
(B) Electrical only
(C) A combination of chemical and electrical events
(D) Mechanical only
(E) None of the above

101. The highest density of cholinergic innervation of any brain structure is found in the

(A) cerebral cortex
(B) caudate nucleus and putamen
(C) cerebellum
(D) spinal cord
(E) locus ceruleus

102. Biological rhythms—cyclic, internally regulated bodily responses—are operative in all the following EXCEPT

(A) birth rate
(B) death
(C) body temperature
(D) personality disorders
(E) depression

103. Deprivation of REM sleep is associated with which of the following?

(A) Onset of psychosis
(B) Dementia-like syndrome
(C) Improvement in depression
(D) Development of personality disorders
(E) Onset of acute anxiety

104. Most studies suggest that the major inhibitory neurotransmitter in the brain is

(A) serotonin
(B) dopamine
(C) beta-endorphin
(D) γ-aminobutyric acid
(E) somatostatin

105. True statements concerning cataplexy include which of the following?

(A) Cataplexy is associated with unconsciousness
(B) Cataplexy involves sudden loss of muscle tone
(C) Cataplexy is unrelated to emotional states
(D) Cataplexy can last up to an hour
(E) Cataplexy is best treated with neuroleptics

106. The highest prevalence of tardive dyskinesia has been observed in

(A) elderly females
(B) young females
(C) elderly males
(D) young males
(E) male and female infants

107. Hypothalamic function is closely related to all the following EXCEPT

(A) sleep
(B) appetite
(C) memory
(D) sexual behavior
(E) fear

108. In the normal adult, the sleep state that constitutes the longest part of the total sleep cycle is

(A) the REM stage
(B) stage 1
(C) stage 2
(D) stage 3
(E) stage 4

109. In the absence of other symptoms, sporadically occurring behavioral automatisms and olfactory hallucinations suggest the diagnosis of

(A) schizophrenia
(B) schizophreniform psychosis
(C) hysterical personality disorder
(D) nondominant parietal lobe lesion
(E) temporal lobe lesion

110. Which of the following neurotransmitters is believed to be associated with the signs and symptoms of opiate withdrawal?

(A) Serotonin
(B) Norepinephrine
(C) Glycine
(D) Acetylcholine
(E) Dopamine

111. The onset of muscular rigidity, tremors, and bradykinesia in a patient being treated with an antipsychotic medication most likely would be due to

(A) Parkinson's disease
(B) increased serotonergic transmission
(C) inhibition of gamma motor neurons
(D) blockage of dopamine receptors
(E) tardive dyskinesia

112. All the following chemical substrates act as neurotransmitters in the brain EXCEPT

(A) dopamine
(B) norepinephrine
(C) 5-hydroxytryptamine
(D) γ-aminobutyric acid
(E) 5-hydroxyindoleacetic acid ·

113. Which of the following types of studies offers the most promise in elucidating the interaction between genetic and environmental factors in psychiatric illness?

(A) Family risk studies
(B) Twin studies
(C) Adoption studies
(D) Genetic marker studies
(E) Prospective longitudinal studies

114. Which of the following pairs of compounds mediates neurotransmission in the greatest number of central nervous system synapses?

(A) Norepinephrine and dopamine
(B) Serotonin and histamine
(C) γ-Aminobutyric acid and glycine
(D) Acetylcholine and norepinephrine
(E) Glutamic acid and serotonin

115. The dietary amino-acid precursor of catecholamines is

(A) tryptophan
(B) glutamic acid
(C) aspartic acid
(D) tyrosine
(E) glycine

DIRECTIONS: Each question below contains four suggested responses of which **one or more** is correct. Select

A	if	**1, 2, and 3**	are correct
B	if	**1 and 3**	are correct
C	if	**2 and 4**	are correct
D	if	**4**	is correct
E	if	**1, 2, 3, and 4**	are correct

116. Studies used to determine the genetic influence in emotional disorders include

(1) twin studies
(2) studies of adoptees and their families
(3) studies of familial risk
(4) studies of drug responses in family members

117. The reticular core includes

(1) noradrenergic pathways
(2) serotonergic pathways
(3) dopaminergic pathways
(4) cholinergic pathways

118. During the last month, a 42-year-old woman who is recently widowed has displayed a markedly dysphoric mood, has lost 6.8 kg (15 lb), has been extremely lethargic, and has experienced vaguely suicidal thoughts. She is in good physical health and has had no previous psychiatric contact. The type of medication most likely to be chosen for the treatment of this woman is thought to act by

(1) increasing postsynaptic receptor sensitivity to serotonin
(2) decreasing plasma levels of dopamine-β-hydroxylase
(3) blocking norepinephrine uptake into synaptic terminals
(4) blocking the accumulation of dopamine at synapses

119. Beta-endorphin is

(1) a substance involved in perception of pain
(2) released from the pituitary in response to stress
(3) a neurotransmitter
(4) a peptide

120. When compared with the general population, relatives of persons who have bipolar affective disorder are more likely to display

(1) alcoholism
(2) antisocial personality
(3) cyclothymic personality
(4) obsessive compulsive personality

121. Investigators attempting to identify biochemical receptors in the central nervous system have discovered receptors to

(1) benzodiazepines
(2) imipramine
(3) opiates
(4) haloperidol

122. Evidence supporting the dopamine hypothesis of schizophrenia includes which of the following observations?

(1) Butyrophenones have molecular configurations similar to those of dopamine
(2) Thioxanthenes can produce parkinsonian side effects
(3) Phenothiazines block dopamine receptors
(4) Antipsychotic medications increase levels of dopamine metabolites

123. True statements about Huntington's disease include which of the following?

(1) It is the result of an autosomal dominant transmission
(2) Significant neuronal loss occurs in the caudate nucleus
(3) A polymorphic DNA marker maps to human chromosome 4 and is linked to the Huntington's disease gene
(4) Dysfunction of brain noradrenergic neurons appears to be the primary pathology

124. Enzymes that are important in the degradation of catecholamines include

(1) catechol-O-methyltransferase
(2) dopa decarboxylase
(3) monoamine oxidase
(4) tryptophan hydroxylase

125. The actions of dextroamphetamine (d-amphetamine) at catecholaminergic synapses include

(1) direct release of catecholamines into the synaptic cleft
(2) blockade of postsynaptic catecholamine receptors
(3) blockade of the catecholamine reuptake mechanism
(4) increased production of catecholamines through an increase in tyrosine hydroxylase

SUMMARY OF DIRECTIONS

A	B	C	D	E
1,2,3	1,3	2,4	4	All are
only	only	only	only	correct

126. Which of the following factors would more likely be associated with antisocial persons than with normal peers?

(1) A history of antisocial behavior in a monozygotic twin
(2) A parent with a criminal record
(3) A history of antisocial behavior in a dizygotic twin
(4) Electroencephalographic abnormalities

127. The Klüver-Bucy syndrome, produced in monkeys by bilateral temporal lobe lesioning, is characterized by

(1) compulsive oral activity
(2) rage attacks
(3) hypersexuality
(4) hypophagia

128. The principal dopaminergic pathway in the brain directly involves which of the following regions of the brain?

(1) Pontine raphe nuclei
(2) Putamen
(3) Locus ceruleus
(4) Substantia nigra

129. Enzymes that are important in the synthesis of catecholamines include

(1) catechol-O-methyltransferase
(2) tyrosine hydroxylase
(3) tryptophan hydroxylase
(4) dopamine-β-hydroxylase

130. The right (nondominant) cerebral hemisphere is thought to mediate or control the function of

(1) visuospatial organization
(2) logical reasoning
(3) perception of body image
(4) quantitative ability

131. REM sleep has been associated with which of the following behavioral and electrophysiological events?

(1) Decreased firing of the dorsal raphe nucleus
(2) Increased muscular activity
(3) Decreased firing of the locus ceruleus
(4) Sleepwalking

132. Persons treated with a monoamine oxidase inhibitor, such as tranylcypromine sulfate (Parnate), for depression show an increase in the functional synaptic availability of

(1) acetylcholine
(2) serotonin
(3) histamine
(4) norepinephrine

DIRECTIONS: Each group of questions below consists of lettered headings followed by a set of numbered items. For each numbered item select the **one** lettered heading with which it is **most** closely associated. Each lettered heading may be used **once, more than once, or not at all.**

Questions 133–136

For each chemical classification, select the CNS neurotransmitter that is an example of that classification.

(A) Glutamic acid
(B) γ-aminobutyric acid
(C) Norepinephrine
(D) Somatostatin
(E) Lactic acid

133. Biogenic amine

134. Excitatory amino acid

135. Neuropeptide

136. Inhibitory amino acid

Questions 137–141

For each function described below, select the hypothalamic nucleus most likely responsible.

(A) Anterior
(B) Ventromedial
(C) Lateral
(D) Posterior
(E) Supraoptic

137. Acts as a satiety center for appetite

138. Stimulates appetite

139. Functions with the reticular activating system to control arousal

140. Influences sexual behavior

141. Produces antidiuretic hormone

Human Behavior: Biological and Related Sciences
Answers

100. The answer is C. *(Michels, vol 3, chap 42, pp 2, 3.)* In the human brain, electrical impulses trigger chemical events. The release of presynaptic neurotransmitters stimulates postsynaptic receptors, allowing neuronal transmission to proceed. Synaptic communication between neurons is primarily chemical, which allows for the continuation of electrical impulses.

101. The answer is B. *(Talbott, pp 16–20.)* The highest density of cholinergic innervation is found in the caudate nucleus and putamen. Acetylcholinesterase-reactive neuronal cell bodies located in the basal forebrain send cholinergic innervation to the cerebral cortex, hippocampus, and limbic structures. The locus ceruleus is the principal noradrenergic nucleus.

102. The answer is D. *(Michels, vol 3, chap 59, pp 1–5.)* Studies have reported that natural births are roughly a third more common at 3 AM than at 5 AM, and deaths 30 percent more common at 5 AM than at midnight. The timing of these events is thought to be directly related to biological rhythm. Body temperature follows a 24-hour rhythm, peaking at midafternoon. Depression has been linked to changes in the cortisol cycle. Personality disorders have not, to date, been linked to any biological rhythm.

103. The answer is C. *(Michels, vol 3, chap 60, pp 12–13.)* Although reports in the early 1960s suggested deprivation of REM sleep as a cause of psychosis and anxiety, this is no longer believed to be true. Deprivation of REM sleep has not been shown to cause any psychopathologic symptoms in recent sleep studies. In fact, 50 percent of depressed patients "tested" with deprivation of REM sleep improved with no other treatment.

104. The answer is D. *(Hales, pp 74–76.)* γ-Aminobutyric acid (GABA) is believed to be the major inhibitory neurotransmitter in the central nervous system. It has an important role in modulating the activity of other neurotransmitters. Many investigators believe that it has an important role in the etiology of anxiety disorders, though the exact mechanisms are still speculative.

105. The answer is B. *(Michels, vol 2, chap 52, p 8.)* Cataplexy is the inability to carry out voluntary muscle movements while awake. It results from a sudden inhibition of muscle tone and varies from complete powerlessness to involvement of isolated muscle groups. It is frequently triggered by intense emotional states and lasts seconds to minutes. Neuroleptics are not used in its treatment.

106. The answer is A. *(Kaplan, ed 4. p 644. Michels, vol 1, chap 55, pp 24–25.)* Tardive dyskinesia is a repetitive involuntary muscle movement of the lips, tongue, jaw, neck, back, or extremities that is seen in some patients late in the course of treatment with antipsychotic medications. It often appears days to weeks after drug treatment is stopped. Its highest prevalence is seen in elderly females.

107. The answer is C. *(Kaplan, ed 4. pp 19–21.)* Lesioning and stimulation studies have shown that the hypothalamus exerts control over sleep, appetite, and sexual and emotional behavior. Hypothalamic hormones and other blood-borne factors can influence behavior; moreover, the release and action of these substances are affected by the neurotransmitters—norepinephrine, serotonin, and dopamine—that mediate behavior. Memory is a complex function that involves cortical and subcortical structures and is affected by hypothalamic activity only in a secondary way.

108. The answer is C. *(Kaplan, ed 4. pp 558–560.)* Stage 2 sleep constitutes about 50 percent of total sleep time. It is characterized by a low-amplitude, fast-frequency electroencephalographic pattern and sleep spindles of 12 to 16 cycles per second. REM sleep accounts for 20 to 25 percent of total sleep time; stages 3 and 4 for 20 percent; and stage 1 for 5 to 10 percent.

109. The answer is E. *(Hales, pp 213–214.)* Temporal lobe lesions are associated with symptoms that can mimic psychiatric illness. These symptoms include affective states (such as anger or depression), depersonalization, and memory impairment. Because olfactory or gustatory hallucinations are relatively rare in psychiatric disorders, their presence should suggest organic disease. Automatisms are complex, stereotyped behaviors carried out during psychomotor seizure activity.

110. The answer is B. *(Kaplan, ed 4. p 394.)* Opiate withdrawal has been shown to be associated with increases in both the firing rate of the locus ceruleus, the major norepinephrine nucleus in the brain, and the concentration of 3-methoxy-4-hydroxyphenylglycol (MHPG), the major metabolite of brain norepinephrine. Moreover, when the drug clonidine is given in doses that decrease brain norepinephrine function, the symptoms of opiate withdrawal in methadone addicts have been successfully treated. Clonidine is thought to affect adrenergic receptors in the locus ceruleus.

111. The answer is D. *(Kaplan, ed 4. p 199.)* Antipsychotic medications are associated with extrapyramidal side effects, such as dyskinesia, akathisia, and symptoms similar to those of Parkinson's disease. These side effects are thought to result from the blockade of dopamine receptors by the antipsychotic medications. The blockade, by causing a *functional* reduction in dopamine, produces a clinical picture similar to that of Parkinson's disease, which is associated with an *actual* dopamine deficiency from degeneration of dopamine neurons.

112. The answer is E. *(Kaplan, ed 4. pp 20–24.)* The list of substances that mediate the transmission of nerve impulses at brain synapses is a growing one. Among the most well-known brain neurotransmitters are dopamine, norepinephrine, 5-hydroxytryptamine (serotonin), and γ-aminobutyric acid (GABA). 5-Hydroxyindoleacetic acid is a metabolite of serotonin.

113. The answer is E. *(Kaplan, ed 4. pp 9–11.)* Prospective longitudinal studies are studies in which persons who are "vulnerable" (i.e., at high risk for psychiatric illness because of a positive family history) are identified at birth and followed over a period of time. Such studies are less subject to methodological bias than other approaches. For example, when compared with retrospective studies, prospective longitudinal studies tend to give a more accurate representation of early signs and symptoms of a given disorder and thus offer a better opportunity for the discovery of successful preventive approaches.

114. The answer is C. *(Kaplan, ed 4. p 19.)* Dopamine, serotonin, and norepinephrine, three of the most intensively studied neurotransmitters in the brain, actually act as transmitters at only a small number of central nervous system synapses. γ-Aminobutyric acid is thought to mediate transmission at 25 to 40 percent of synapses in various regions of the brain. Amino acids, including glycine, serve as neurotransmitters in a significant percentage of synapses in the spinal cord and brain.

115. The answer is D. *(Kaplan, ed 4. p 22.)* The amino acid tyrosine is the precursor in the synthesis of dopamine and norepinephrine. Tyrosine is converted to 3,4-dihydroxyphenylalanine (dopa), which is then decarboxylated to dopamine. Through the action of the enzyme dopamine-β-hydroxylase, dopamine is converted to norepinephrine. According to current biochemical theories, this pathway is of critical importance in the pathogenesis of depression.

116. The answer is A (1, 2, 3). *(Kaplan, ed 4. pp 9–11.)* In determining the genetic influence in emotional disorders a variety of research models have been employed. Following twins through their lives, particularly when they are identical twins, is the most common method. Most research centers maintain twin registries. Studies of adoptees are valuable in determining nature versus nurture issues, as are studies of familial risk. Drug responses are not used in determining genetic factors.

117. The answer is E (all). *(Talbott, pp 16–17.)* The reticular core is believed to be highly involved in the pathophysiology of major mental illness. It appears to modulate neuronal function in wide areas of the nervous system, with influences on drives, affects, arousal and cognitive functions. The associated noradrenergic, cholinergic, serotonergic and dopaminergic pathways have been widely studied in psychiatry.

118. The answer is B (1, 3). *(Kaplan, ed 4. pp 25–26.)* The woman described in the question most likely has a retarded depression and should have been treated with a tricyclic antidepressant. The exact mechanism of action of this class of medication is not known but is thought to involve inhibition of the reuptake of norepinephrine, dopamine, and serotonin. Recent studies also have shown that chronic administration of these drugs increases postsynaptic receptor sensitivity to norepinephrine and serotonin.

119. The answer is E (all). *(Talbott, pp 8–9.)* The endorphins are endogenous opioid peptides that are highly distributed in the brain. Their discovery led to the identification of a number of peptides that are thought to serve as neurotransmitters. Beta-endorphin has aroused considerable interest in psychiatry since it is released by the pituitary in response to stress and has an important role in perception of pain.

120. The answer is A (1, 2, 3). *(Kaplan, ed 4. p 127.)* Family studies of persons with documented bipolar affective disorders have shown a higher-than-expected frequency of relatives who are alcohol abusers or who display antisocial behavior or cyclic mood variation. In general, the morbidity is higher for relatives of persons with bipolar disease than for relatives of persons with unipolar disease. Family history of obsessive compulsive personality does not appear to affect morbidity in or increase the incidence of bipolar affective illness.

121. The answer is A (1, 2, 3). *(Talbott, pp 10–11.)* Psychopharmacologists, using specific radioactive ligands, have identified benzodiazepine, opiate, and imipramine receptors in the brain. These findings prompted speculation about whether endogenous substances exist that interact with these receptors. Endogenous opiate substances subsequently were identified, and the search for endogenous antianxiety and antidepressant compounds continues.

122. The answer is E (all). *(Kaplan, ed 4. pp 198–199.)* The hypothesis that schizophrenic symptoms are associated with abnormalities of dopamine metabolism is based on the fact that all effective antipsychotic medications block dopamine receptors. Such blockade results in increased production of dopamine (but decreased functional availability) and correspondingly increased levels of dopamine metabolites. Similarities in the molecular configurations of antipsychotic drugs and dopamine have been demonstrated by x-ray crystallography. Symptoms of Parkinson's disease, a disorder associated with dopamine deficiency in the brain, are produced as side effects of many antipsychotic medications.

123. The answer is A (1, 2, 3). *(Kaplan, ed 4. p 14. Nemeroff, Science 221:972–973, 1983.)* Huntington's disease is inherited as an autosomal dominant trait. Neuropathological and radiological observations indicate significant neuronal loss in the caudate nucleus. Neurochemical changes associated with Huntington's disease include decreased activity of glutamic acid decarboxylase, choline acetyltransferase, and cysteic acid decarboxylase and decreases in the concentration of γ-aminobutyric acid (GABA). There are reduced numbers of brain membrane receptors for cholecystokinin, quinuclidinyl benzoate, benzodiazepines, haloperidol, dopamine, GABA, and kainic acid. Increased brain levels of neurotensin, somatostatin, and thyrotropin-releasing hormone have been identified. No specific abnormalities in brain noradrenergic function have been observed. A recent study using molecular genetic techniques that involve enzymes that cleave DNA into distinct "restriction fragment length polymorphisms" has identified a DNA marker on chromosome 4 that is linked to Huntington's disease.

124. The answer is B (1, 3). *(Kaplan, ed 4. pp 22–23.)* Catecholamines are degraded by two primary enzymes. Catechol-*O*-methyltransferase methylates norepinephrine and intermediate metabolites. Monoamine oxidase deaminates norepinephrine and normetanephrine to their corresponding aldehydes. One class of antidepressant agents acts by inhibition of monoamine oxidase. Tryptophan hydroxylase is an enzyme involved in the synthesis of serotonin, and dopa decarboxylase is involved in catecholamine synthesis.

125. The answer is B (1, 3). *(Kaplan, ed 4. p 24.)* Dextroamphetamine is a drug with mood-stimulating and appetite-suppressing properties. These properties are thought to be related to *d*-amphetamine's capacity to increase the synaptic availability of catecholamines by releasing them directly into synapses and by blocking their reuptake. The *dextro* isomer of amphetamine is three to four times as potent a stimulant of the central nervous system as the *levo* isomer.

126. The answer is E (all). *(Kaplan, ed 4. pp 856–858.)* Current evidence supports the notion that both genetic and experiential factors are important in the development of antisocial personality disorder. Twin-family studies of antisocial behavior have shown higher concordance rates in monozygotic than in dizygotic twins, though rates in dizygotic twins still are higher than in controls. Antisocial parents have been found to have a greater risk of producing antisocial offspring. Antisocial personality disorder is associated with an increased frequency of electroencephalographic abnormalities.

127.   The answer is B (1, 3). *(Kaplan, ed 4. p 780.)* The Klüver-Bucy syndrome occurs in monkeys following bilateral temporal lobectomy involving the amygdala, the parahippocampal gyrus, the hippocampus, and the temporal cortex. It is a syndrome characterized by psychic blindness, compulsive oral activity, docility, hypersexuality, hyperphagia, and inability to ignore stimuli. Bilateral temporal lobe lesions in humans can produce modified versions of the same symptoms as well as severe memory loss.

128.   The answer is C (2, 4). *(Michels, vol 3, chap 44, pp 6–8.)* Neuroanatomical and neurochemical studies have revealed the presence of several dopaminergic pathways in the brain. The principal pathway has its origins in the substantia nigra and terminates in the caudate nucleus and putamen of the corpus striatum. Degeneration of this pathway causes the symptoms of Parkinson's disease. Other dopaminergic pathways originate in the cerebral cortex, arcuate nucleus of the hypothalamus, and in an area of the brain just dorsal to the interpeduncular nucleus.

129.   The answer is C (2, 4). *(Kaplan, ed 4. p 22.)* Enzymes that are important in the synthesis of catecholamines include the following: tyrosine hydroxylase, which converts tyrosine to 3,4-dihydroxyphenylalanine (dopa); dopa decarboxylase, which converts dopa to dopamine; and dopamine-β-hydroxylase, which converts dopamine to norepinephrine. Understanding this series of reactions is important in defining the role of catecholamines not only in psychiatric disorders but in other clinical situations as well. (For example, L-dopa is the preferred treatment of Parkinson's disease, and α-methyldopa is a commonly used medication in the treatment of hypertension.)

130.   The answer is B (1, 3). *(Kaplan, ed 4. p 681.)* Studies of persons with unilateral brain lesions as well as of persons who have had cerebral commissurotomies have suggested that the right cerebral hemisphere mediates certain nonverbal modes of perception and performance. In contrast to the left hemisphere, which is thought to control verbal, logical, and mathematical processes, the right hemisphere is thought to mediate visuospatial organization, perception of part-whole relationships, perception of rhythm, and integration of sensory and kinesthetic stimuli to form body images. Sex, age, and handedness can modify the asymmetry of cerebral hemispheric function.

131.   The answer is B (1, 3). *(Kaplan, ed 4. pp 242, 558.)* REM sleep—also known as D-sleep—is the stage of sleep in which dreaming occurs. Electrophysiological studies have found that the firing rates of both the locus ceruleus and the dorsal raphe decrease markedly with the onset of REM sleep. Sleepwalking occurs during stage 4 sleep and thus is not associated with dreaming.

132.   The answer is C (2, 4). *(Kaplan, ed 4. pp 657–660. Michels, vol 1, chap 61, p 11.)* Tranylcypromine sulfate (Parnate) is a member of the class of antidepressant drugs known as monoamine oxidase (MAO) inhibitors. Because the enzyme MAO is involved in the catabolism of both norepinephrine and serotonin, inhibition of this enzyme increases the availability of these neurotransmitters.

133–136. The answers are: 133-C, 134-A, 135-D, 136-B. *(Hales, p 59.)* CNS neurotransmitters include amino acids, biogenic amines, and neuropeptides. There are many other neurotransmitter substances, and many are still poorly understood. This is one of the most exciting areas of current psychiatric research. As more and more knowledge accrues, it becomes possible to develop more specific psychopharmacologic interventions. The amino acids are excitatory (glutamic acid, aspartic acid) or inhibitory (GABA). The biogenic amines include the catecholamines such as dopamine, norepinephrine, and epinephrine. Other biogenic amines include acetylcholine, histamine, and the indolamine serotonin. There are numerous neuropeptides, including beta-endorphin, somatostatin, and vasopressin.

137–141. The answers are: 137-B, 138-C, 139-D, 140-A, 141-E. *(Kaplan, ed 4. pp 19, 20, 517. Michels, vol 1, chap 28, p 7.)* The hypothalamus plays a central role in regulating a variety of physiological functions that directly affect behavior and thus is key to the biological expression of psychiatric illness. Sleep, appetite, and sexual and aggressive behavior are subject to its control. In addition, the hypothalamus regulates temperature, fluid balance, and pituitary function.

Through electrical stimulation and ablation studies, hypothalamic nuclei have been identified as having defined functions. The anterior nucleus appears to facilitate sexual interest and specific sexual behavior; lesions in this area eliminate the behavior. The ventromedial nucleus acts as a satiety center; stimulation of this area reduces appetite. The ventromedial nucleus exerts its control through inhibition of the lateral nucleus, which stimulates appetite. Ablation of the lateral nucleus results in fatal anorexia regardless of the state of the ventromedial nucleus. The posterior nucleus along with the contiguous reticular activating system controls the level of arousal; lesions in this area result in lethargy and somnolence. Aggression appears to be affected by stimulation of a number of different hypothalamic sites.

The hypothalamus also exerts control over the pituitary gland. The supraoptic and paraventricular hypothalamic nuclei produce vasopressin (antidiuretic hormone) and oxytocin, respectively. These hormones traverse the axons of their parent neurons to the posterior pituitary gland, from which they are released. The hypothalamus also produces a variety of releasing factors that control hormone secretion from the anterior pituitary gland.

Organic Mental Disorders and Consultation-Liaison Psychiatry

DIRECTIONS: Each question below contains five suggested responses. Select the **one best** response to each question.

142. All the following statements about complex partial seizures are true EXCEPT

(A) they are also known as psycho-motor or temporal lobe seizures
(B) impaired consciousness or loss of contact with the environment occurs
(C) the patient remembers associated automatisms as uncontrollable events
(D) associated automatisms can be ictal or postictal
(E) the focus is in temporal (limbic) structures

143. When assessing depression in the medically ill, which of the following symptoms is frequently the most diagnostic?

(A) Sleep disorder
(B) Poor appetite
(C) Low self-esteem
(D) Low energy level
(E) Decreased sex drive

144. The primary gain in a conversion disorder is the

(A) resolution of the conflict-related anxiety
(B) lack of responsibility for the associated symptoms
(C) exclusion from everyday responsibilities
(D) attention given by the physician
(E) attention given by the family

145. All the following statements about absence seizures are true EXCEPT

(A) they are also known as petit mal
(B) they are associated with an abrupt loss of attention to the environment
(C) the patient does not usually show confusion following the episode
(D) the loss of consciousness is usually for between 1 and 2 minutes
(E) during a seizure the patient may stare blankly or show automatisms such as lip smacking

146. Normal-pressure hydrocephalus is associated with the clinical triad of

(A) dementia, visual hallucinations, and seizures
(B) dementia, gait disturbance, and incontinence
(C) personality changes, gait disturbance, and aphasia
(D) personality changes, seizures, and incontinence
(E) none of the above

147. A 32-year-old woman complains of left-hand anesthesia, which developed after an argument with her husband. There is no history or evidence of trauma or other neurological abnormalities. The likely diagnosis is

(A) hysteria
(B) histrionic personality
(C) conversion disorder
(D) psychogenic fugue
(E) none of the above

148. The occurrence of delusions de novo in a person over the age of 35 years and without a known history of schizophrenia or delusional disorder should always alert the diagnostician to the possibility of

(A) agoraphobia
(B) frotteurism
(C) sleep disorder
(D) substance abuse
(E) dissociative disorder

149. Huntington's chorea is associated with all the following EXCEPT

(A) autosomal dominant inheritance
(B) chromosomal abnormalities
(C) cerebral atrophy
(D) personality changes
(E) onset during adulthood

150. In which of the following age groups is the incidence of psychopathology the greatest?

(A) Under 10 years
(B) 10 to 25 years
(C) 25 to 45 years
(D) 45 to 65 years
(E) Over 65 years

151. A man given a placebo for mild pain reports 30 minutes later that the pain has resolved. The most appropriate conclusion is that the man

(A) has a conversion disorder
(B) has a dissociative disorder
(C) is malingering
(D) had no real pain to begin with
(E) responds to placebos

152. A 62-year-old woman is admitted to a medical unit because of an 11.4-kg (25-lb) weight loss over the last 3 months. She also reports anorexia, insomnia, fatigue, and decreased sexual interest. She does not have depressed affect and her mental status is judged to be unimpaired. Extensive medical evaluation is unremarkable. The most likely diagnosis is

(A) senile dementia
(B) occult malignancy
(C) hypochondriasis
(D) chronic anxiety
(E) masked depression

153. The most common cause of dementia in the elderly is

(A) multiple cerebral infarcts
(B) normal pressure hydrocephalus
(C) Alzheimer's disease
(D) Huntington's disease
(E) hardening of cerebral arteries

154. The sudden loss of muscular strength in association with laughter is most consistent with which of the following conditions?

(A) Catatonia
(B) Epilepsy
(C) Cataplexy
(D) Narcolepsy
(E) Hysteria

155. Organic mental disorders typically are characterized by

(A) mental confusion, disorientation, and memory loss
(B) mental confusion, auditory hallucinations, and thought disorder
(C) depression, auditory hallucinations, and disorientation
(D) depression, visual hallucinations, and thought disorder
(E) depression, grandiosity, and sleep disorder

156. The most common psychiatric disturbance associated with Cushing's syndrome is

(A) depression
(B) psychosis
(C) organic mental disorder
(D) mania
(E) anxiety neurosis

DIRECTIONS: Each question below contains four suggested responses of which **one or more** is correct. Select

A	if	**1, 2, and 3**	are correct
B	if	**1 and 3**	are correct
C	if	**2 and 4**	are correct
D	if	**4**	is correct
E	if	**1, 2, 3, and 4**	are correct

157. Symptoms commonly associated with premenstrual syndrome include

(1) irritability
(2) anxiety
(3) tension
(4) depression

158. Clinical observations of familial emotional responses in the premenstruum show that

(1) girls tend to repeat the symptom patterns of their mothers
(2) symptoms tend to peak in the fourth decade of life
(3) 5 to 10 percent of all women experience severe symptoms
(4) when daughters leave their mother's home, symptoms cease

159. Patients with organic mental syndromes commonly have symptoms involving

(1) behavior
(2) personality
(3) emotion
(4) cognition

160. The syndrome of delirium is usually characterized by

(1) inattention
(2) depressed affect
(3) clouded consciousness
(4) garrulousness

161. Correct statements about chronic subdural hematomas include which of the following?

(1) The majority are caused by head trauma
(2) The most common symptom is headache
(3) The symptoms may progress over days to weeks
(4) Fluctuations of consciousness predominate over any focal or lateralizing signs

162. The "epileptic personality" of patients with temporal lobe seizure commonly includes

(1) hyperreligiosity
(2) hypersexuality
(3) circumstantiality
(4) panic attacks

Questions 163–165

A 52-year-old man presents with the chief complaint of feelings of hopelessness and helplessness, loss of interest, and poor sleep for the past 3 weeks. He is 25 lb overweight and smokes a pack of cigarettes a day. One month ago he was started on antihypertensives for his moderate hypertension of 150/95. He reports being fired from his job of 18 years 6 weeks ago.

163. This patient's differential diagnosis should include

(1) adjustment disorder with depressed mood
(2) organic mood syndrome
(3) major depression
(4) dysthymia

164. Appropriate management of his hypertension should include

(1) a weight reduction program
(2) a reduction of salt intake
(3) a regular exercise program with smoking reduction
(4) a rechecking of his blood pressure

165. If this patient began complaining of impotence, the likely causes would include

(1) drug effect
(2) primary impotence
(3) stress
(4) penile steal syndrome

166. Psychiatric features of Addison's disease include

(1) depression
(2) memory impairment
(3) irritability
(4) psychosis

167. Cluster headaches tend to differ from migraine in that they

(1) have no known precipitants
(2) are more common in males than females
(3) are often associated with agitation and at times head banging
(4) display a very slow onset with a typical prodromal phase

168. The condition known as sleep apnea is characterized by

(1) reduced stage 3 and stage 4 sleep
(2) loud snoring
(3) excessive daytime sleepiness
(4) episodic cessation of breathing during sleep

169. Subcortical dementias include

(1) Huntington's disease
(2) Parkinson's disease
(3) Wilson's disease
(4) Alzheimer's disease

170. In primary degenerative dementia of the Alzheimer type

(1) the onset is abrupt
(2) the onset is usually after the age of 65 years
(3) the loss of intellectual abilities is limited to memory functions
(4) there are changes in personality and behavior

171. Catatonia may be a feature of which of the following conditions?

(1) Mania
(2) Alcoholism
(3) Epilepsy
(4) Schizophrenia

172. Features that commonly distinguish multi-infarct dementia from dementia of the Alzheimer type include

(1) a stepwise deterioration in intellectual functioning ("patchy" deterioration)
(2) an abrupt onset
(3) focal neurologic signs and symptoms
(4) an absence of personality changes

173. A normal grief reaction typically involves

(1) guilt feelings about neglecting the deceased
(2) anger toward physicians
(3) somatic distress
(4) residual depression a year later

174. Night terrors differ from nightmares in which of the following ways?

(1) They affect children more often than adults
(2) They are associated with marked autonomic changes
(3) They are difficult to remember
(4) They are associated commonly with psychological disturbances in children

175. The Kleine-Levin syndrome is a disorder characterized by

(1) periodic attacks of hypersomnolence
(2) an onset usually in adolescence
(3) gluttony and hypersexuality during the episode
(4) a higher incidence in males

176. Acute intermittent porphyria is characterized clinically by which of the following?

(1) Abdominal pain
(2) Constipation
(3) Psychosis
(4) Neurological deficits

177. Elisabeth Kubler-Ross has described five major phases that occur in a person's psychological adjustment to impending death. These stages include

(1) acceptance
(2) denial
(3) anger
(4) bargaining

178. True statements regarding the hyperventilation syndrome include that it

(1) is usually associated with severe anxiety
(2) may be caused by salicylism, fever, and pulmonary emboli
(3) is associated with respiratory alkalosis
(4) may induce paresthesias, numbness, and tetany

179. Medications that can produce depression include

(1) reserpine
(2) imipramine
(3) prednisone
(4) insulin

180. Klüver-Bucy syndrome is a neurological condition characterized by

(1) visual agnosia
(2) hypersexuality
(3) hyperorality
(4) unilateral deafness

181. People who have Munchausen's syndrome characteristically

(1) have factitious medical illnesses
(2) are pursuing disability
(3) wander from hospital to hospital
(4) downplay their medical histories

182. An 82-year-old man who is hospitalized for evaluation of hematuria is noted to be depressed and is started on a tricyclic antidepressant. Toxicity from the tricyclic antidepressant would be likely to affect this man's

(1) kidneys
(2) brain
(3) lungs
(4) heart

183. Subcortical arteriosclerotic encephalopathy is associated with

(1) hypertension
(2) white matter lesions
(3) dementia
(4) seizures

184. A 55-year-old man, who is taking lithium carbonate for manic-depressive illness, is admitted to a hospital because of cardiac disease. Which of the following therapeutic measures might be expected to increase the man's plasma lithium concentration even if his lithium dosage remains constant?

(1) Administration of digitalis
(2) Administration of a thiazide diuretic
(3) Administration of methyldopa
(4) Maintenance on a low-sodium diet

DIRECTIONS: Each group of questions below consists of lettered headings followed by a set of numbered items. For each numbered item select the **one** lettered heading with which it is **most** closely associated. Each lettered heading may be used **once, more than once, or not at all.**

Questions 185–188

Match the following.

(A) Wernicke's encephalopathy
(B) Korsakoff's psychosis
(C) Huntington's disease
(D) Wilson's disease
(E) Creutzfeldt-Jakob disease

185. Rapidly progressive and fatal dementia with a usual age of onset in the forties or fifties

186. An abrupt onset with oculomotor disturbances, cerebellar ataxia, and mental confusion

187. A chronic condition that characteristically presents with confabulation and memory problems

188. A disorder characterized by choreiform movements and dementia, with an age of onset usually in the thirties

Questions 189–195

For each concept in "psychosomatic medicine" below, select the name that is most closely associated with it.

(A) Elisabeth Kubler-Ross
(B) Franz Alexander
(C) Sigmund Freud
(D) Wilhelm Reich
(E) Flanders Dunbar

189. Psychosomatic illnesses are associated with specific unresolved neurotic conflicts

190. There are seven psychosomatic illnesses: bronchial asthma, ulcerative colitis, rheumatoid arthritis, essential hypertension, peptic ulcer disease, neurodermatitis, and Graves' disease

191. Hysterical neurosis results from memories that have been repressed

192. Psychosomatic illnesses are characterized by specific personality traits

193. Persons experiencing life-threatening illness go through distinct stages of psychological adjustment

194. Psychoanalysis should address the underlying character type as well as symptoms

195. Hysterical (i.e., histrionic) personality is characterized by seductiveness, excitability, and superficial interpersonal relationships

DIRECTIONS: The group of questions below consists of four lettered headings followed by a set of numbered items. For each numbered item select

A	if the item is associated with	(A) **only**
B	if the item is associated with	(B) **only**
C	if the item is associated with	**both** (A) and (B)
D	if the item is associated with	**neither** (A) nor (B)

Each lettered heading may be used **once, more than once, or not at all.**

Questions 196–198

(A) Premenstrual syndrome (PMS)
(B) Dysmenorrhea
(C) Both
(D) Neither

196. Symptoms most prominent in the late luteal phase

197. Antipsychotic medication indicated in treatment

198. Symptoms affected by diet and exercise

Organic Mental Disorders and Consultation-Liaison Psychiatry

Answers

142. The answer is C. *(Hales, pp 213–214.)* Impairment of consciousness is a hallmark of complex partial seizures. The focal discharge is associated with a temporal aura, and as this discharge spreads to the limbic system impaired consciousness and loss of contact with the environment ensue. Automatisms are highly integrated, unconscious movements not remembered by the patient. They commonly include such activities as lip smacking, rubbing, running, disrobing or the perseveration of acts initiated prior to loss of consciousness. Automatisms can be ictal or postictal events.

143. The answer is C. *(Michels, vol 2, chap 120, pp 2–3.)* Patients with medical illness can develop many of the vegetative signs of depression—for example, sleep problems, decreased appetite, low energy, and decreased sexual interest—as a result of being ill and in the hospital. In these patients the cognitive-affective symptoms, or how one feels about oneself, are commonly the most important diagnostic cues.

144. The answer is A. *(Michels, vol 2, chap 95, pp 12–13.)* Conversion disorders represent psychological conflicts expressed as physical symptoms or signs. The primary gain associated with a conversion disorder is the minimization of anxiety, achieved by resolving the psychological conflict through the expression of signs or symptoms. Being excused from everyday responsibilities and the attracting of extra attention are examples of secondary gain.

145. The answer is D. *(Hales, p 214.)* During an absence seizure, also called petit mal, the patient has an abrupt loss of attention while remaining awake and maintaining posture. The seizure activity rarely lasts beyond 20 seconds, and the patient displays an abrupt return of attention without residual confusion. Stereotyped or automatic behavior (such as lip smacking, chewing, or blinking) is common, but there is not a generalized convulsion. Some patients may show mild clonic, atonic, or tonic activity.

146. The answer is B. *(Kaplan, ed 4. p 306.)* Although many dementias are chronic, slowly progressive, and unresponsive to specific treatment, one notable exception is the dementia associated with normal-pressure hydrocephalus. This dementia may be difficult to diagnose but often is precipitated by such acute events as subarachnoid hemorrhage, trauma, or meningitis. It is associated with gait disturbances and urinary incontinence. A dramatic clinical improvement can be effected by shunting cerebrospinal fluid away from the central nervous system and into the cardiovascular system.

147. The answer is C. *(Kaplan, ed 4. pp 342–348.)* The probable diagnosis for the woman presented in the question is conversion disorder. The anesthesia of her left hand represents the somatic expression of an intrapsychic conflict. Psychogenic fugue is associated with unexpected travel away from home, inability to recall one's past, and assumption of a new personal identity. The diagnosis of histrionic personality refers to a life-style characterized by dramatic behavior, dependency, difficulty in delaying gratification, and shallow interpersonal relationships. The term *hysteria* often is used pejoratively to mean that a person's symptoms are not real; hysteria is not an actual diagnosis.

148. The answer is D. *(American Psychiatric Association, ed 3-R. pp 109–110.)* Schizophrenia and delusional disorder most often, but not always, first appear in persons under the age of 35 years. When delusions appear de novo without such a history, one must always consider the possibility of an organic delusional disorder. Abuses of substances such as cannabis, cocaine, amphetamines, and hallucinogens are common causes of organic delusional syndrome. Other causes include cerebral lesions and interictal phenomena in temporal lobe epilepsy.

149. The answer is B. *(Kaplan, ed 4. p 14.)* Huntington's chorea is a rare illness that is inherited as an autosomal dominant trait and typically manifests during adulthood. It is characterized clinically by choreiform movements, dementia, and personality changes. No effective treatment is presently known. At autopsy, the brain of affected persons is atrophied, especially in the caudate nucleus and putamen. Chromosomal abnormalities are not associated with Huntington's chorea.

150. The answer is E. *(Kaplan, ed 4. pp 881–884.)* Persons older than 65 years of age have a higher risk than other persons of developing mental illness. However, elderly persons are underrepresented in the frequency of visits to mental-health clinics and in the receipt of appropriate social services. Common psychiatric problems in this population include depression and organic mental disorders.

151. The answer is E. *(Michels, vol 3, chap 45, pp 8–9.)* The only conclusion that can be reached about the man described in the question is that he responds to placebos. His response says nothing about whether his pain is "real" or psychogenic.

Placebos have been shown to decrease pain of both psychological and physiological origin.

152. The answer is E. *(Michels, vol 1, chap 59, p 12.)* Depressive illness consists of both somatic and psychological components. The somatic components include insomnia, anorexia, weight loss, fatigue, motor retardation or agitation, and decreased sexual interest. The psychological components include depressed mood, pessimism, and feelings of worthlessness and guilt. Not all components are present in every case. Patients who have a masked depression present with primarily somatic symptoms and few or no psychological ones. Diagnosis often is made only after extensive medical evaluation is unrevealing. The woman described in the question did not have any signs of dementia; medical evaluation did not reveal an organic disease process; and although hypochondriasis and chronic anxiety could have caused many of her symptoms, they are not likely to have caused the 11.4-kg weight loss.

153. The answer is C. *(Michels, vol 1, chap 73, pp 5–8.)* Although estimates vary, it is currently believed that 50 percent of demented elderly suffer from senile dementia of the Alzheimer type. The cause of this disorder is unknown and no treatment for it exists. Approximately 20 percent of demented elderly suffer from cerebral arteriosclerosis (previously described as hardening of the cerebral arteries). Cerebral arteriosclerosis produces dementia by causing multiple cerebral infarcts. Normal pressure hydrocephalus and Huntington's disease are rare causes of dementia.

154. The answer is C. *(Kaplan, ed 4. p 177.)* Cataplexy is the sudden and brief loss of muscular tone that occurs during the expression of a strong emotion. Affected persons remain conscious throughout each episode, which usually lasts no longer than 2 minutes. Cataplexy often occurs in patients with narcolepsy who may also have hypnagogic phenomena and sleep paralysis. The cause is unknown.

155. The answer is A. *(Kaplan, ed 4. pp 272, 273.)* An organic mental disorder is characterized by disorientation, memory loss, mental confusion, and occasionally by visual hallucinations. The disorder occurs commonly in both medical and surgical patients and is often the result of metabolic abnormalities or adverse reactions to medication. When the disorder has an acute onset, reversible causes should be sought.

156. The answer is A. *(Kaplan, ed 4. pp 517–518.)* Cushing's syndrome often is associated with psychiatric disturbances. Depression is the most common disturbance and may range from moderate to severe; as many as 10 percent of affected persons attempt suicide. Mania, psychosis, and an organic mental disorder also can occur.

157. The answer is E (all). *(Michels, vol 2, chap 120, p 2.)* There have been many physical and emotional symptoms associated with premenstrual syndrome

(PMS). Irritability, tension, depression, and anxiety are among the most common. Physical symptoms include breast tenderness, abdominal bloating, and swelling of the ankles. Some researchers have attempted to cluster certain symptoms together in an attempt to delineate PMS subtypes. The reliability of this is questionable.

158. The answer is A (1, 2, 3). *(Michels, vol 2, chap 120, p 2.)* Clinical observation of menstrual responses in families has shown a tendency for girls to repeat the symptom patterns of their mothers. These do not change when leaving home. Symptoms of the premenstrual syndrome tend to peak in the fourth decade of life. It is estimated that approximately 5 to 10 percent of women in the United States experience severe menstrual symptoms.

159. The answer is E (all). *(Nicholi, pp 358–360.)* Patients with organic mental disorders often display defects of cognitive function. This is demonstrated on the mental status examination by difficulties with memory, calculation, language, and proverb interpretation. However, often there are also changes in noncognitive functions such as behavior, personality, and emotional regulation. Personality change and the appearance of lack of emotional control should always alert the clinician to the possibility of this diagnosis.

160. The answer is B (1, 3). *(Nicholi, pp 360–363.)* Delirious states usually have a sudden onset, often in the context of a medical illness. The most common finding is a defect in attention. This presents as an inability to concentrate, as well as distractibility. The patient is often unable to complete a coherent sentence and may misperceive distracting stimuli. Disorientation and memory loss may be present, but are not essential to the diagnosis. The disturbance of consciousness may extend from quietness and a tendency to fall asleep all the way to lethargy, stupor, or coma. Some patients display hypervigilance or agitation or have illusions or hallucinations.

161. The answer is E (all). *(Hales, pp 195–196.)* Approximately 60 percent of chronic subdural hematomas follow head trauma. Other causes include ruptured aneurysms and rapid deceleration injuries. Headache is the most common symptom. As increased intracranial pressure gradually increases, one encounters signs associated with dementia. These include confusion, inattention, apathy, memory loss, drowsiness, and ultimately coma. Fluctuations in the level of consciousness predominate over focal or lateralizing neurological signs, though such signs are not rare.

162. The answer is B (1, 3). *(Hales, p 218.)* The so-called epileptic personality described for patients with temporal lobe seizures commonly includes hyperreligiosity, circumstantiality, and hypergraphia. These patients most commonly display hyposexuality. On the MMPI they often have elevations on the paranoia and schizophrenia scales. It is important to remember that all of these psychiatric manifestations can occur in other psychiatric disorders.

163–165. The answers are: 163-A (1, 2, 3), 164-E (all), 165-B (1, 3). *(American Psychiatric Association, ed 3-R. pp 112, 222–223, 232–233, 330–331.)* In assessing this patient's symptoms we find a significant stressor—losing a job of 18 years—which could account for an adjustment disorder. He is taking antihypertensive medication, which may be associated with the onset of depressive feelings (i.e., an organic mood syndrome). Since his dysphoria has lasted for longer than 2 weeks, and since he also has loss of interest in past pleasurable activities, as well as poor sleep, major depression cannot be ruled out. Dysthymia is not a consideration, since this diagnosis requires a 2-year history of depressive symptoms.

Nondrug measures used in the treatment of hypertension include relief of stress, dietary management, regular exercise, and control of other risk factors, such as cigarette smoking. Dietary management involves the restriction of sodium, cholesterol, and saturated fats, as well as the restriction of calories if the patient is overweight. Regular monitoring of blood pressure is indicated.

Male impotence, the inability to obtain or maintain an erection, or the inability to achieve orgasm, can be brought on by a variety of biological, psychological, or social causes. Antihypertensive medications are notorious for causing impotence, as is emotional stress. Primary impotence is when a man never had normal sexual functioning. The penile steal syndrome occurs when blood is diverted from the penis to the gluteal region with resultant detumescence.

166. The answer is E (all). *(Kaplan, ed 4. p 517.)* Addison's disease results from atrophy of the adrenal cortices. This may result from primary degeneration or be secondary to other diseases such as tuberculosis. The production of adrenal steroids is greatly diminished. Common psychiatric features include depression, apathy, anxiety, and irritability. Memory impairment may occur in as many as three-fourths of patients. Although rare, psychosis may also be present.

167. The answer is A (1, 2, 3). *(Hales, pp 226–230.)* Cluster headaches share some similarities with migraine, but they also have some distinguishing features. The female-to-male ratio is 2:3, as opposed to 3:1 for migraine. There are usually flurries of attacks, without a known precipitant. The onset is generally rapid and severe. Migraine usually has a more gradual onset, but both types of headache may be associated with nausea and vomiting. Migraine patients usually want to lie still, since movement aggravates their pain. Cluster headache patients are often agitated and may even bang their head in an effort to relieve pain.

168. The answer is E (all). *(Kaplan, ed 4. pp 568, 569.)* Sleep apnea is a chronic and generally progressive syndrome characterized by episodic cessation of breathing during sleep and loud snoring due to partial airway obstruction. Because this condition interrupts sleep and reduces both stage 3 and stage 4 sleep, it often produces severe daytime sleepiness. The syndrome can occur in children as well as adults. Its cause is unknown, although hereditary factors appear to be involved.

169. The answer is A (1, 2, 3). *(Kaplan, ed 4. pp 276, 277. Michels, vol 1, chap 73, p 10.)* Subcortical dementias involve the basal ganglia, thalamus, and rostral brainstem structures. Because of this, these dementias have movement disorders as a prominent part of their symptoms. Typical examples include Huntington's disease, Parkinson's disease, and Wilson's disease. In contrast, Alzheimer's disease represents a type of cortical dementia that does not involve subcortical structures and does not manifest a movement disorder.

170. The answer is C (2, 4). *American Psychiatric Association, ed 3-R. pp 119–120.)* In primary degenerative dementia of the Alzheimer type there is an insidious onset with a progressive and deteriorating course. The dementia involves multiple areas of cognition, including memory, judgment, abstract thinking, and other higher cortical functions. There are often profound changes in personality and behavior as the disorder progresses.

171. The answer is E (all). *(Michels, vol 2, chap 95, p 6.)* Catatonia is characterized by waxy flexibility, posturing, mutism, facial grimacing, and negativism. Though generally considered to occur only in schizophrenic persons, it is actually a nonspecific syndrome. In fact, catatonia has occurred in association with mania, alcoholism, epilepsy, and head trauma, as well as with schizophrenia.

172. The answer is A (1, 2, 3). *(American Psychiatric Association, ed 3-R. pp 121–122.)* Multi-infarct dementia is due to cerebrovascular disease and is usually associated with focal neurologic signs and symptoms. The onset is typically abrupt, with a stepwise course that early on may leave some intellectual functions relatively intact. The deficits are "patchy" depending on which areas of the brain are damaged. In Alzheimer's dementia the onset is more gradual, and the course more uniformly progressive. Both conditions are associated with significant personality and behavioral changes.

173. The answer is A (1, 2, 3). *(Kaplan, ed 4. pp 264–266.)* Grief reactions typically occur in the close relatives of a deceased person. Normal grief reactions are characterized by guilt feelings, thoughts about the deceased, somatic distress, anger toward physicians, and disorganized behavior. Usually the various manifestations, including depression, last 1 to 4 months. Characteristics of abnormal grief reactions include delayed onset, adoption of the symptoms of the deceased, and extremely irrational behavior. A small proportion of grief reactions are abnormally prolonged and develop into serious depressive illnesses that require treatment.

174. The answer is A (1, 2, 3). *(Kaplan, ed 4. pp 572–573.)* Night terrors occur more commonly in children than in adults and are characterized by extreme anxiety, marked autonomic changes, and vocalizations. Nightmares are much more common than night terrors, occur in persons of all ages, are less frightening, and are associated with only slight autonomic changes. Persons experiencing nightmares are more easily aroused and better able to recall the content of their dreams. Although both persistent nightmares and night terrors may be associated with evidence of psychopathology in adults, only persistent nightmares seem to be linked with psychopathology in children.

175. The answer is E (all). *(Hales, p 253.)* Kleine-Levin syndrome is a disorder of sleep. It is characterized by periodic attacks of hypersomnolence and megaphasia. Most often it has an onset in adolescence, more commonly in males, but it may begin later in life. Hypersexuality and personality disturbances are also seen during episodes. Sleepiness may be as severe as that seen in narcolepsy or obstructive sleep apnea, and sleep studies often show multiple sleep-onset REM periods.

176. The answer is E (all). *(Kaplan, ed 4. pp 309, 310.)* Abdominal pain, constipation, neurological deficits, and psychosis are all clinical features of acute intermittent porphyria. Although the course of the disease is extremely variable, initial presentation often consists of recurrent attacks of abdominal pain, with neurological and emotional disturbances developing later. Attacks of the illness may be precipitated by medication, especially barbiturates. The diagnosis can be established by testing urine for porphobilinogen.

177. The answer is E (all). *(Kaplan, ed 4. p 586.)* Elisabeth Kubler-Ross has described five phases of psychological adjustment that people pass through when confronted with the knowledge they are dying. Characteristically, the first state involves denial of death and isolation of feelings. Affected persons then experience anger at their fate and may begin bargaining (often with God) in order to avert death. A period of depression finally is followed by acceptance. These responses do not necessarily occur in this sequence; several of them may occur simultaneously, or they may be mixed with other responses.

178. The answer is E (all). *(Talbott, pp 502–503.)* Hyperventilation leads to decreased arterial P_{CO_2}, increased pH, and resultant respiratory alkalosis. It is usually associated with severe anxiety. The cause may be anxiety or any medical condition that can produce hyperventilation. Such conditions include salicylism, fever, and pulmonary emboli. Patients usually complain of light-headedness, numbness around the lips, or tingling sensations in the extremities. Tetany occurs if the condition becomes severe.

179. The answer is B (1, 3). *(Kaplan, ed 4. p 509.)* Depression is often present in people who have a physical illness. Although it usually represents a psychological reaction to the illness itself, depression can be associated with medical disease for other important reasons. For example, in certain illnesses, such as retroperitoneal neoplasms, hypothyroidism, and hyperparathyroidism, depression may be a prominent clinical feature. In addition, certain medications, such as reserpine and corticosteroids, can produce depression, which often recedes when the dosage is decreased or the medication is stopped altogether. Insulin and imipramine (an antidepressant) do not precipitate depression.

180. The answer is A (1, 2, 3). *(Kaplan, ed 4. p 780.)* The Klüver-Bucy syndrome is a behavioral syndrome following destructive lesions to both temporal lobes. Conditions that produce the syndrome include viral encephalitis, trauma, infarction, Pick's disease, and Alzheimer's disease. This behavioral syndrome is characterized by visual agnosia (e.g., inability to distinguish relatives from strangers), hypermetamorphosis (e.g., manual exploration of the environment), hyperorality (i.e., bulimia, or placing nonfood items in mouth), hypersexuality, aphasia, amnesia, and dementia. The hyperorality and hypersexuality may superficially resemble the behavior of patients suffering from mania.

181. The answer is B (1, 3). *(Kaplan, ed 4. pp 552–554.)* People who have Munchausen's syndrome wander from hospital to hospital presenting a dramatic medical history. The history, which may be totally fictitious, is usually bolstered by artificially produced signs and symptoms of acute medical illness, such as fever, seizures, or hemorrhage. Affected persons are pursuing gratification from being a patient. In contrast, malingering patients utilize fictitious medical signs and symptoms to pursue specific goals (e.g., disability compensation, lawsuits, exemption from military duty).

182. The answer is C (2, 4). *(Kaplan, ed 4. pp 650–657.)* Prominent side effects and adverse reactions to tricyclic antidepressants include orthostatic hypotension, cardiac arrhythmias, and mental confusion. All these effects are especially likely in older persons, who commonly tolerate orthostatic hypotension poorly, who often have underlying cardiac disease, and who may also have a mild organic mental disorder. Occasionally, a toxic psychosis occurs because of the drugs' strong anticholinergic activity. In therapeutic dosages, tricyclic antidepressants have little or no effect on the renal and respiratory systems.

183. The answer is A (1, 2, 3). *(Michels, vol 1, chap 73, p 10.)* Subcortical arteriosclerotic encephalopathy is a condition associated with hypertension that affects the deep perforating arteries supplying the periventricular white matter. In its severe form it is diagnosed as Binswanger's disease, a variant of multi-infarct dementia affecting white matter. This condition is being diagnosed more frequently with the advent of x-ray computed tomography and magnetic resonance imaging of the head. Seizures are not associated with this condition.

184. The answer is C (2, 4). *(Kaplan, ed 4. p 675, 676.)* Lithium carbonate is eliminated from the body through urinary excretion. Both low-sodium diets and use of thiazide diuretics increase lithium concentrations in the plasma by increasing the reabsorption of lithium by the kidney. Thus, patients placed on either or both of these treatments should have their plasma concentration of lithium frequently monitored and the dosage of lithium adjusted accordingly to avoid toxicity.

185–188. The answers are: 185-E, 186-A, 187-B, 188-C. *(Hales, pp 119, 149–152.)* Both Wernicke's and Korsakoff's syndromes are associated with thiamine deficiency, often resulting from alcoholism. Wernicke's encephalopathy has an abrupt onset with mental confusion, cerebellar ataxia, and oculomotor disturbances such as nystagmus or gaze palsy. The general confusional state may ultimately deteriorate, with the development of Korsakoff's psychosis and ultimately stupor and coma. Korsakoff's psychosis is chronic, with both retrograde and anterograde amnesia. Confabulation is common.

Creutzfeldt-Jakob disease may present with neurotic-like symptoms or as dementia and is fatal. It usually begins in the forties or fifties and rapidly progresses to severe dementia and death often in 1 year. It appears to be caused by a "slow" virus.

Wilson's disease is due to an inborn error of copper metabolism and usually has an onset in adolescence. The early onset with bizarre behavior and flattened affect may lead to a misdiagnosis of schizophrenia, although the neurological signs usually precede the psychiatric symptoms. Not all cases show significant psychiatric symptoms.

Huntington's disease is a hereditary disorder that usually begins when the patient is in his or her late thirties. It is associated with choreiform movements and a progressive dementia that eventually, over decades, culminates in apathy and death.

189–195. The answers are: 189-B, 190-B, 191-C, 192-E, 193-A, 194-D, 195-D. *(Kaplan, ed 4. pp 66, 108, 268, 489.)* Sigmund Freud developed the concepts of psychological conflict and repression. He believed that persons who had hysterical neuroses suffered from the repression of memories and the feelings associated with them. His original ideas led to the development of psychoanalysis and laid the groundwork for psychosomatic medicine. Freud's early work was concerned mainly with symptoms.

Wilhelm Reich, a student of Freud, called attention to the importance of character types in diagnosis and treatment. One of the personality types he discussed was the hysterical personality, which he characterized as seductive, easily excitable, and superficial in interpersonal relationships.

Personality type and psychological conflict both have been cited as pathogenetic factors causing physical symptoms and psychosomatic illnesses. Flanders Dunbar thought that persons who had psychosomatic illnesses had specific personality traits. Franz Alexander gave major impetus to the concept that the seven classic psychosomatic illnesses—bronchial asthma, ulcerative colitis, rheumatoid arthritis, essential hypertension, peptic ulcer disease, neurodermatitis, and Graves' disease—were characterized by specific, unresolved neurotic conflicts. For example, he felt that persons with peptic ulcer disease had conflicts about oral dependency. Recent investigators, however, have questioned the specificity of his formulations, in part because many neurotic conflicts occur in association with more illnesses than the seven listed by Alexander. In fact, most—if not all—medical and surgical illnesses have concomitant psychological factors; in that sense, they are all psychosomatic in nature.

Elisabeth Kubler-Ross has written extensively on psychological adjustment to impending death.

196–198. The answers are: 196-A, 197-D, 198-C. *(Michels, vol 2, chap 120, pp 2–3.)* Premenstrual syndrome (PMS) is characterized by the onset of symptoms, both physical (breast tenderness, abdominal swelling) and emotional (irritability, depression, anxiety) in the late luteal phase, usually the week before the onset of menses. The patient is symptom-free during the first 2 weeks after her menstrual period starts. Dysmenorrhea is pain associated with the time of menstrual flow, usually the first 2 or 3 days. Mild analgesics, particularly nonsteroidal anti-inflammatory agents, are used for dysmenorrhea. Both conditions can be improved with exercise and dietary manipulation. PMS has responded to anxiolytics like alprazolam, but not antipsychotics.

Schizophrenia, Delusional, and Other Psychotic Disorders

DIRECTIONS: Each question below contains five suggested responses. Select the **one best** response to each question.

199. Which of the following statements regarding thought disorder is true?

(A) It is invariably found in schizophrenia

(B) It is sometimes exhibited by patients with mania

(C) It is one of the main criteria for the diagnosis of schizophrenia in the third edition of *Diagnostic and Statistical Manual of Mental Disorders (DSM III-R)*

(D) It is reflected in the speech but not the written communication of schizophrenics

(E) It is a phenomenon of schizophrenia first described by Sigmund Freud

200. Which of the following statements regarding delusions is true?

(A) Delusions are almost exclusively found in schizophrenia

(B) Delusions of grandiosity are rarely encountered except in mania

(C) Delusions involve a disturbance of cognition

(D) Delusions involve a disturbance of perception

(E) Delusions are a type of hallucination

201. Chronic schizophrenic patients who display smacking or sucking movements of their lips and tongue

(A) probably are suffering from tardive dyskinesia

(B) are usually undermedicated with neuroleptics

(C) have cerebellar lesions

(D) have the hebephrenic form of the disorder

(E) will often lose these symptoms under the influence of rehabilitative and resocialization therapies

202. Studies of schizophrenic persons who had been adopted as infants have shown that

(A) the incidence of schizophrenia in their biological parents is the same as in the general population
(B) the degree of psychopathology in their adoptive parents is significantly higher than in the general population
(C) environmental factors have no major role in the etiology of schizophrenia
(D) there is a genetic predisposition to schizophrenia
(E) adoption per se encourages the development of schizophrenia

203. Schizotypal personality disorder (formerly known as latent schizophrenia) is a term used to describe people who have

(A) a strong predisposition to becoming schizophrenic
(B) bizarre styles of communicating or thinking
(C) overt delusions and hallucinations
(D) onset of schizoprenia late in life
(E) no family history of schizophrenia

204. Which of the following signs or symptoms would best discriminate a person with an organic brain syndrome from a person with schizophrenia?

(A) Confusion
(B) Tangential thinking
(C) Auditory hallucinations
(D) Visual hallucinations
(E) Gradual onset of symptoms

205. Which of the following drugs may induce a psychosis that is easily confused with, or misdiagnosed as, paranoid schizophrenia?

(A) Barbiturates
(B) Heroin
(C) Benzodiazepines
(D) Amphetamines
(E) Chlorpromazine

206. Evaluation of which of the following would be LEAST helpful in reaching a prognosis for a schizophrenic patient?

(A) Marked auditory hallucinations
(B) Work history
(C) Closeness of interpersonal relationships
(D) History of hospitalizations
(E) Prior level of social functioning

207. The first major studies on the psychological features of schizophrenia were done by

(A) Anna Freud
(B) Carl Jung
(C) Eugen Bleuler
(D) Kurt Schneider
(E) Sigmund Freud

208. The lifetime risk for suicide in schizophrenic patients is estimated to be approximately

(A) 0.5 percent
(B) 3 percent
(C) 10 percent
(D) 25 percent
(E) 35 percent

209. Among schizophrenic patients maintained on neuroleptic medication for 1 year after hospitalization, the proportion that can be expected to experience psychotic relapse

(A) is about 5 percent
(B) is about 30 percent
(C) is about 55 percent
(D) is about 80 percent
(E) cannot be specified because it will depend to a large extent on whether the medication is given in oral or long-acting injectable form

210. In the criteria set forth by *DSM III-R,* which of the following would distinguish schizophrenia from a manic episode?

(A) The schizophrenic patient will exhibit evidence of a thought disorder
(B) The manic patient is persistently elated, whereas the schizophrenic patient displays blunted, flat, or inappropriate affect
(C) The schizophrenic's psychosis is most often treated with neuroleptic medication
(D) The schizophrenic's psychosis is chronic while manic episodes are always intermittent
(E) None of the above

211. Correct statements regarding the diagnostic criteria for delusional (paranoid) disorder, according to *DSM III-R,* include all the following EXCEPT

(A) auditory or visual hallucinations, if present, are not prominent
(B) behavior is not bizarre
(C) delusions are bizarre
(D) any associated affective syndrome is of brief duration relative to the duration of the delusional disturbance
(E) an organic factor has not initiated and maintained the disturbance

212. The diagnosis of schizoaffective disorder includes all the following EXCEPT

(A) the condition does not meet the criteria for schizophrenia
(B) the condition does not meet the criteria for mood disorder
(C) the patient has presented with both schizophrenic psychotic symptoms and a mood disturbance, and at other times with psychotic symptoms without mood symptoms
(D) during an episode there have been delusions or hallucinations for at least 2 days but less than 2 weeks
(E) no organic factor initiated or maintained the disturbance

DIRECTIONS: Each question below contains four suggested responses of which **one or more** is correct. Select

A	if	**1, 2, and 3**	are correct
B	if	**1 and 3**	are correct
C	if	**2 and 4**	are correct
D	if	**4**	is correct
E	if	**1, 2, 3, and 4**	are correct

213. True statements about the course and prognosis of schizophrenia include which of the following?

(1) Some schizophrenic illnesses will resolve completely and never recur, even without treatment
(2) Outcome has improved considerably in the last 50 years
(3) Catatonic and hebephrenic forms have become less frequent
(4) Research suggests an initial onset following a stressful event may be associated with a better prognosis

214. True statements about the occurrence of thought disorder include which of the following?

(1) Bleuler considered it the most important characteristic of schizophrenia
(2) It occurs frequently in schizophrenia and affective disorders
(3) Its presence may cause manic patients to be misdiagnosed as schizophrenic
(4) It disappears when the patient is no longer actively psychotic

215. The *DSM III-R* criteria for schizophreniform disorder include

(1) all the psychotic symptom criteria for schizophrenia except for duration
(2) schizophrenic-like symptoms caused by hallucinogens
(3) an illness that lasts less than 6 months
(4) severe affective symptoms with thought disorder but no other signs of schizophrenia

216. Correct statements regarding paranoid disorders include that they

(1) are more common than schizophrenia
(2) are associated with delusions that are usually less bizarre and fragmented than in schizophrenia
(3) are associated with delusions of persecution, but not of jealousy
(4) usually are not associated with Schneiderian first-rank symptoms

217. The use of neuroleptics to manage and treat schizophrenia may be associated with which of the following side effects?

(1) Acute dystonia
(2) Gynecomastia
(3) Parkinsonism
(4) Galactorrhea

218. Signs or symptoms more likely to be associated with the catatonic type of schizophrenia than with other subtypes include

(1) neologisms
(2) psychomotor disturbance
(3) word salad
(4) excitement and stupor

219. Correct statements about malignant neuroleptic syndrome include that it is

(1) believed to result from blockade of dopamine receptors in the brain
(2) characterized by severe autonomic and extrapyramidal dysfunction
(3) associated with hyperthermia
(4) usually fatal

220. The relationship between lower socioeconomic status and higher prevalence rates of schizophrenia

(1) has been attributed to the downward social mobility of schizophrenic persons
(2) has been attributed to the conditions within lower socioeconomic environments that foster social isolation
(3) is supported by prevalence rates in lower socioeconomic populations even twice those found in higher socioeconomic groups
(4) is found in both rural and urban settings

221. Some researchers have divided symptoms of schizophrenia into negative and positive. Negative symptoms include

(1) hallucinations
(2) blunted affect
(3) delusions
(4) social withdrawal

222. The thought disorder of schizophrenic persons usually consists of marked disturbance of

(1) memory
(2) logic
(3) orientation
(4) abstraction

DIRECTIONS: Each group of questions below consists of lettered headings followed by a set of numbered items. For each numbered item select the **one** lettered heading with which it is **most** closely associated. Each lettered heading may be used **once, more than once, or not at all.**

Questions 223–225

Match the following.

(A) Invalidation
(B) Pseudomutuality
(C) Schism
(D) Fragmented communication
(E) Skew

223. An overt conflict that hides covert dependence within a marriage

224. An overt harmony coupled with covert hostility within a marriage

225. The family acting as a system to maintain a rigid equilibrium

Questions 226–229

Match the following.

(A) Emil Kraepelin
(B) Eugen Bleuler
(C) Harry Stack Sullivan
(D) Frieda Fromm-Reichman
(E) Sigmund Freud

226. The schizophrenogenic mother

227. Dementia praecox renamed to schizophrenia

228. Interpersonal theory of schizophrenia

229. The symptoms of schizophrenia (dementia praecox) delineated on the basis of course and outcome

Schizophrenia, Delusional, and Other Psychotic Disorders

Answers

199. The answer is B. *(Michels, vol 1, chap 53, pp 9–12.)* The abnormalities found in schizophrenic speech and writing were originally best described by Kraepelin and Bleuler. While these were originally considered to be a hallmark of that illness, modern investigation and clinical experience have shown that they can also be exhibited by patients with other psychiatric disorders, such as mania. Thought disorder is commonly found in schizophrenia, but there are significant numbers of patients who do not demonstrate the phenomenon. *DSM III-R* recognizes that a disturbance in thinking is but one of a number of criteria that are necessary to make the diagnosis.

200. The answer is C. *(Talbott, p 365.)* Delusions are found in a wide variety of psychotic conditions other than schizophrenia, including organic disorders and some mood disorders. A delusion is defined as a firmly held belief that is untrue and contrary to a person's educational and cultural background. The patient clings to the belief even in the face of great contrary evidence. The delusions of schizophrenia show a wide variety of themes, but no particular theme is specific to either schizophrenia or any other mental disorder. While grandiose delusions are a common finding in mania, they are also found in other conditions. Hallucinations are disorders of perception.

201. The answer is A. *(Michels, vol 1, chap 53, p 14.)* A large number of chronic schizophrenic patients will display the characteristic smacking or sucking movements of their lips and tongue associated with the syndrome of tardive dyskinesia. It is presumed that this is a consequence of neuroleptic medication, especially with long-term use. Some patients may also have involuntary movements of other parts of the body, such as choreoathetoid movements of the limbs. It is hypothesized that the mechanism involves supersensitivity of postsynaptic dopamine receptors.

202. The answer is D. *(Michels, vol 1, chap 62, pp 4–12.)* Investigators have been able to separate to some degree the contributions of environment and heredity to the etiology of schizophrenia by studying schizophrenic persons who were adopted as infants. The adoptive parents in these studies showed only minimally more psychopathology than a matched sample of parents whose adopted children did not grow up to be schizophrenic. The studies did reveal, however, that there was a higher level of schizophrenia in the biological relatives of the adoptees than in the general population, thus pointing to a genetic predisposition for the disorder.

203. The answer is B. *(American Psychiatric Association, ed 3-R. pp 340–342. Michels, vol 1, chap 16, pp 4–8.)* Schizotypal personality disorder is a new diagnostic category that has replaced latent schizophrenia. It defines a group of socially isolated nonpsychotic persons who have bizarre modes of thought and patterns of communication. They are often eccentric and suspicious. Although chronic schizophrenia appears to occur more commonly in relatives of persons with schizoptypal personality disorder than in the general population, there is no evidence to suggest that this disorder predisposes a person to develop schizophrenia later in life.

204. The answer is D. *(Kaplan, ed 4. pp 558, 681–691.)* Because visual hallucinations are unusual in association with schizophrenia, their occurrence in persons having a psychotic illness should raise the suspicion of an organic brain syndrome. Visual hallucinations in schizophrenic persons tend to be as common during the day as at night; however, in persons with an organic brain syndrome, visual hallucinations occur more frequently at night. Auditory hallucinations, confusion, tangential thinking, and gradual onset of symptoms are highly characteristic of schizophrenia but also can occur in association with organic brain syndromes.

205. The answer is D. *(Nicholi, pp 270–271.)* Abuse of amphetamines can result in a psychosis very closely resembling acute paranoid schizophrenia. Symptoms include paranoid delusions and visual hallucinations. Some investigators feel that prominent visual hallucinations and a relative absence of thought disorder are more characteristic of amphetamine psychosis, but other investigators feel the symptoms are indistinguishable. Other drugs that produce psychoses similar to schizophrenia include phencyclidine (PCP) and lysergic acid diethylamide (LSD).

206. The answer is A. *(Kaplan, ed 4. pp 709–712. Strauss, pp 57–67.)* In general, prognosis is better judged by past performance than by the characteristics of the schizophrenic patient at the time of diagnosis. Some of the better prognostic indicators available for schizophrenic patients include their work histories, number of hospitalizations, closeness of interpersonal relationships, and previous levels of social participation. Illnesses that develop acutely in response to stress will in general have a better prognosis than those that develop insidiously.

207. The answer is C. *(Kaplan, ed 4. pp 680–681. Strauss, pp 1–7.)* Eugen Bleuler coined the term schizophrenia in 1911 for the disorder that formerly had been called dementia praecox by Emil Kraepelin. In the course of his work, Bleuler took the cluster of clinical phenomena that previously had been observed in association with dementia praecox and weighted each symptom as of either primary or secondary importance in the overall clinical picture of schizophrenia. In 1930, he first referred to the "four A's" of schizophrenia: association, affect, autism, and ambivalence. Although this concept is not as widely used for diagnosis today as in the past, Bleuler's work focused diagnostic attention on observable psychological features associated with schizophrenia.

208. The answer is C. *(Stoudemire, pp 220–221.)* The lifetime risk for suicide in schizophrenic patients is estimated at 10 percent. This is somewhat less than is the case for mood disorders. Alcoholics have a similar lifetime risk, estimated at 12 percent.

209. The answer is B. *(Michels, vol 1, chap 55, pp 5–7.)* Over the past 2 decades, studies have agreed that about 30 percent of schizophrenic patients will relapse into psychosis despite maintenance on neuroleptic medication. It is clear that neuroleptic maintenance reduces, but does not eliminate, risk of relapse into psychosis. Relapse rates have been similar even in studies in which compliance is controlled through the use of long-acting injectable medications.

210. The answer is E. *(American Psychiatric Association, ed 3-R. pp 192–195, 216–218. Talbott, pp 360–362.)* None of the distinctions set forth in this question apply to the disorders. An affective diagnosis may be associated with "first rank" symptoms such as thought broadcasting or thought insertion; and similarly, the presence of mood-incongruent delusions or hallucinations, in the absence of a full affective syndrome, may point toward schizophrenia. While it is true that in schizophrenia there must be continuous signs of illness for at least 6 months, this need not be continuous psychosis but may include prodromal or residual symptoms. Mania is usually episodic, but chronicity of psychosis does not exclude the diagnosis of mania if other criteria are fulfilled. It is true that most often mania is treated by lithium, but neuroleptic medication is commonly used with both schizophrenia and in the acute phases of mania. Also, treatment methodology is not part of the diagnostic criteria.

211. The answer is C. *(American Psychiatric Association, ed 3-R. pp 201–202.)* The delusions in delusional (paranoid) disorder are not bizarre. This fact helps to differentiate the condition from paranoid schizophrenia or schizophreniform disorder where delusions are usually bizarre and hallucinations are often present. In delusional disorder the delusions usually involve situations that occur in real life, such as being followed, poisoned, loved at a distance, and so on.

212. The answer is D. *(American Psychiatric Association, ed 3-R. pp 209–210.)* The diagnosis of schizoaffective disorder is one of the most confusing and controversial in psychiatric nosology. It is considered when the condition does not meet the criteria for either schizophrenia or mood disorder but at one time has presented with symptoms of both, and, at another time, with psychotic symptoms without mood symptoms. During an episode of the disturbance the delusions or hallucinations must have been present for at least 2 weeks, in the absence of prominent mood symptoms.

213. The answer is E (all). *(Michels, vol 1, chap 53, pp 16–18.)* The outcome of schizophrenic illnesses is very variable, and it has long been known that some will resolve completely, with or without treatment. Other patients will have repeated recurrences, with either full or partial recovery between episodes. Still other patients will show a relentless downhill course. It is clear that prognosis has improved over the years, presumably as a result of better treatment. Paranoid forms of the disorder have become more common, while catatonic and hebephrenic illnesses are less common. A number of studies have demonstrated that there are characteristics of the initial illness that are more likely to be associated with a good prognosis. These include an acute onset following stress, confusion or perplexity, and prominent affective symptoms. However, if schizophrenia is defined as in *DSM III-R,* it may be that these "good prognosis" patients were suffering with affective or schizophreniform disorders.

214. The answer is A (1, 2, 3). *(Talbott, p 365.)* While thought disorder was regarded as the salient symptom of schizophrenia by Bleuler, research has clearly demonstrated that it also occurs in manic and depressive patients. The tangential looseness of associations (derailment) and illogicality of manic patients is also common in schizophrenic patients. There is no specific thought disorder that is exclusively found in schizophrenia. Often the thought disorder will lessen or disappear with the resolution of the active psychosis, but this is by no means a certainty. The thought disorder may continue to be evident even during remission.

215. The answer is B (1, 3). *(Michels, vol 1, chap 70, pp 8–10.)* DSM III-R criteria for schizophreniform disorder meet all the criteria for schizophrenia, except that the duration is less than 6 months. This includes all phases of the disorder, including the prodromal and residual phases. It probably includes many of the cases of "good prognosis schizophrenia" that were described in many early studies of prognosis. By definition these patients do not include those with sufficient affective symptoms to be diagnosed as having an affective disorder, nor patients with drug-induced or other organic psychoses.

216. The answer is C (2, 4). *(Michels, vol 1, chap 68, pp 1–15.)* Paranoid disorders are associated with psychosis that includes persistent delusions of persecution or of jealousy, but lacks the criteria for a diagnosis of schizophrenia, affective disorder, brief reactive disorders, or organic mental disorder. The delusions are typically more "tightly organized" and less bizarre and fragmented than in schizophrenia. It must be remembered that paranoid symptoms may be associated with organic mental disorder, such as that produced by use of amphetamines.

217. The answer is E (all). *(Michels, vol 1, chap 55, pp 20–26.)* Neuroleptic medication is associated with a wide variety of potential side effects. The antidopaminergic drugs may produce a number of extrapyramidal movement disorders, such as dystonias, parkinsonism, tardive dyskinesia, and akasthisia. They may also elevate prolactin levels, which may result in gynecomastia, galactorrhea, and sexual and menstrual dysfunction. Another serious side effect is the potentially fatal malignant neuroleptic syndrome.

218. The answer is C (2, 4). *(American Psychiatric Association, ed 3-R. p 196.)* The essential feature of the catatonic type of schizophrenia is psychomotor disturbance. This may present as stupor, negativism, posturing, rigidity, or excitement. Mutism is common, as is alteration between extreme excitement and stupor. The condition is now relatively rare.

219. The answer is A (1, 2, 3). *(Michels, vol 1, chap 55, p 25.)* Malignant neuroleptic syndrome is a very serious side effect of treatment with neuroleptic medication. It is potentially fatal, with a mortality that approaches 20 percent. Typically there is severe autonomic and extrapyramidal dysfunction, altered consciousness, and hyperthermia. Laboratory findings include leukocytosis and elevated creatine phosphokinase. An early diagnosis and discontinuance of neuroleptics are essential. The response to drugs such as bromocriptine mesylate has suggested that dopamine receptor antagonism is associated with this disorder.

220. The answer is E (all). *(Kaplan, ed 4. pp 667–668.)* Higher incidence and prevalence of schizophrenia have been found repeatedly to occur in association with lower socioeconomic conditions, whether urban or rural. This evidence is, however, more striking in large urban centers than in small cities or rural areas. One investigator, M. L. Kohn, believes that the incidence actually may be as much as six times as high in lower socioeconomic groups as that found elsewhere in society. Whether the relationship between schizophrenia and socioeconomic status is causal (i.e., due to the social isolation characteristic of poor environments) or a result of the downward social drift of schizophrenic persons is controversial; probably both factors contribute to the increased rate.

221. The answer is C (2, 4). *(American Psychiatric Association, ed 3-R. pp 187–198.)* *Schizophrenia* is a term used to represent a group of mental disorders that include such symptoms as delusions, hallucinations, and formal thought disorder. These disorders usually have an onset by early adulthood, though sometimes much later, and may be associated with a deterioration of functioning over time. Some researchers have divided symptoms into positive and negative. Positive symptoms, such as hallucinations and delusions, usually respond to antipsychotic medications. Negative symptoms, such as blunted affect and social withdrawal, are less consistently responsive.

222. The answer is C (2, 4). *(Kaplan, ed 4. pp 658–686.)* Schizophrenic persons tend to have private and unconventional styles of thinking, which appear neither logical nor sensible when verbalized. Interpretation of proverbs is a clinical tool to demonstrate inability to generalize correctly or to use abstraction. The mentation disorders of schizophrenia, unlike those of many organic syndromes, typically do not include severe impairment of memory or orientation.

223–225. The answers are: 223-C, 224-E, 225-B. *(Kaplan, ed 4. pp 735, 1427.)* Frieda Fromm-Reichmann initiated interest in the families of schizophrenic persons through her descriptions of the mothers of affected persons. She used the term *schizophrenogenic* to label those mothers whom she found to be cold, distant, and rejecting. Subsequent investigators have felt that no specific type of psychopathology is characteristic of either or both parents of the schizophrenic person. Instead, these investigators tend to view the entire family as a pathogenic system.

Gregory Bateson and coworkers described a pathogenic family pattern called the *double bind,* in which the preschizophrenic person is expected to respond accurately to mixed messages. Murray Bowen used the term *ego mass* to conceptualize the interdependence of all family members. He felt that a typically disrupted form of ego mass called *emotional divorce* occurs in schizophrenic families. In this situation, parents share the same environment but live in different worlds.

Theodore Lidz also described marital patterns that were characteristic of schizophrenic families. *Schism* was used to describe a marriage in which there was overt conflict but covert dependence; *skew* was used to describe an apparent lack of marital conflict coupled with covert hostility. Lidz believed that the children in such families found their perceptions, feelings, and opinions systematically denied, altered, or ignored through a process called *invalidation.*

Lyman Wynne described a related process termed *pseudomutuality,* in which preschizophrenic people were prevented from breaking out of the roles they were playing in a distorted and rigid family system. Pseudomutuality was seen as a mechanism that maintained role homeostasis, avoided conflicts, and prevented normal separation. Wynne further believed that *fragmented communication* was a typical, deviant mode of communication used by families with schizophrenic members. This mode was thought to reflect the inability of the family to share a common focus of attention.

226–229. The answers are: 226-D, 227-B, 228-C, 229-A. *(Talbott, pp 358–360, 380–381.)* Emil Kraepelin (1828–1899) carefully studied the course and outcome of seriously mentally ill patients. He noted that some had symptoms such as delusions and withdrawal at a relatively early age and were likely to have a chronic and deteriorating course. To distinguish these patients with "dementia" at an early age from those with late-onset dementias, Alzheimer's disease, and manic depressive illness, he referred to the disorder as dementia praecox.

Bleuler (1857–1939) also observed patients over long periods of time and became convinced that a thought disorder, involving a "splitting" of cognitive functions, was the pathognomonic feature of this disorder. He renamed the condition *schizophrenia*.

Sigmund Freud felt that these patients were untreatable by psychoanalysis because of their severe libidinal regression, which made them unable to form relationships, and in particular a transference.

Sullivan saw schizophrenia not so much in intrapsychic terms, but as a result of environmental influence in which the patient had an insufficient developmental exposure to positive interpersonal relationships.

Fromm-Reichman believed that schizophrenia was the outcome of an inadequate mother-child relationship in which the mother was aloof, overly protective, or hostile.

Mood Disorders

230. While the majority of women do not experience significant side effects when taking oral contraceptives, for those who do, the most commonly encountered psychological problem is

(A) anxiety
(B) depression
(C) night terrors
(D) short-term memory defects
(E) long-term memory defects

231. Twin studies of bipolar illness show an average concordance rate in monozygotic twins of

(A) 10 percent
(B) 25 percent
(C) 50 percent
(D) 75 percent
(E) 95 percent

232. One week after the death of her father, a woman describes many memories of her father and says that she is occasionally tearful and is having some trouble falling asleep. She returned to work 4 days after her father's death. Proper treatment for this woman should consist of

(A) antidepressant medication
(B) long-term psychotherapy
(C) referral for further psychiatric evaluation
(D) a longer period of time away from work
(E) brief, supportive treatment

233. The occurrence of depression, as an early symptom, has been particularly associated with carcinoma of the

(A) prostate
(B) bladder
(C) parathyroid
(D) pancreas
(E) ovary

234. A 27-year-old woman seeks evaluation for her "depression" in an outpatient clinic. She reports episodic feelings of sadness since adolescence. Occasionally she feels good, but these periods seldom last more than 2 weeks. She is able to work but thinks she is not doing as well as she should. In describing her problems she seems to focus more on repeated disappointments in her life and her low opinion of herself than on discrete depressive symptoms. In your differential diagnosis at this point, the most likely diagnosis is

(A) major depression with melancholia
(B) adjustment disorder with depressed mood
(C) cyclothymia
(D) childhood depression
(E) dysthymia

235. The cognitive functioning of a person with a major depression is often characterized by all the following manifestations EXCEPT

(A) bizarre associations
(B) suicidal ideation
(C) obsessive rumination
(D) concentration impairment
(E) memory impairment

236. All the following statements about postpartum depression and "maternity blues" are true EXCEPT

(A) postpartum depression occurs in 10 to 15 percent of all new mothers
(B) "maternity blues" occur in 50 to 80 percent of all new mothers
(C) postpartum depression is differentiated from "maternity blues" by persistence beyond the first 3 days following delivery
(D) the signs and symptoms of postpartum depression may be similar to those of a major depressive episode
(E) the treatment of postpartum depression is similar to that for major depression

237. The basis for the therapeutic effect of electroconvulsive therapy (ECT) is

(A) seizure activity
(B) electrical stimulation of the brain
(C) memory loss
(D) the depressed patient's wish for punishment
(E) the depressed patient's attitude toward ECT

238. Among seriously depressed patients, the proportion that can be expected eventually to suicide is

(A) less than 1 percent
(B) about 2 percent
(C) about 15 percent
(D) about 30 percent
(E) about 60 percent

239. All the following statements about suicide are true EXCEPT

(A) it is among the top ten leading causes of death in the United States
(B) it is almost always associated with illness, especially depression
(C) it has a significant familial incidence
(D) it is more apt to be completed in males than in females
(E) it is less likely in persons who have communicated their intent to others

240. A diagnosis of bipolar disorder might be appropriate for patient's who have all the following EXCEPT

(A) recurrent depressions and a history of mania
(B) recurrent depressions without a history of mania
(C) mania now and a history of a depressive episode
(D) mania now without a history of past affective disturbances
(E) a history of several manic episodes without depression

241. According to *DSM III-R*, all the following characteristics are found in the melancholic type of major depressive episode EXCEPT

(A) typically worse depression in the evening
(B) early morning awakening
(C) psychomotor retardation or agitation
(D) significant anorexia or weight loss
(E) loss of interest or pleasure in all or most activities

242. The psychoanalyst associated with the concept that psychopathology, including depression, is the result of developmental deficits related to self-esteem and the development of a cohesive self is

(A) Franz Alexander
(B) Carl Jung
(C) Harry Stack Sullivan
(D) Heinz Kohut
(E) Sigmund Freud

243. Persons having a psychotic major depressive episode most often suffer from delusions that

(A) they are the Messiah
(B) the FBI is out to get them
(C) their sins or misdeeds bring harm to others
(D) they were reborn
(E) they are an unusual animal

244. The term *double depression* is used to describe

(A) a particularly severe bout of major depression
(B) major depression superimposed on dysthymia
(C) recurrent episodes of major depression within a 2-month period
(D) medical illness with a superimposed episode of major depression
(E) major depression superimposed on "maternity blues"

245. According to *DSM III-R*, all the following are criteria for a diagnosis of recurrent major depression EXCEPT

(A) there must have been at least two major depressive episodes
(B) recurrent major depressive episodes must have been separated by a period of at least 1 year of more or less usual functioning
(C) the current episode need not meet the full criteria for a major depressive episode if there has been a previous major depressive episode
(D) there has never been a manic episode
(E) there has never been an unequivocal hypomanic episode

246. All the following statements about bipolar disorder are true EXCEPT

(A) the essential feature is one or more manic episodes usually accompanied by one or more major depressive episodes
(B) the initial episode that occasions hospitalization is usually depression
(C) there may be two or more complete cycles within a year
(D) mixed or rapidly cycling bipolar disorder tends to have a more chronic course than other types
(E) the disorder is equally common in males and females

DIRECTIONS: Each question below contains four suggested responses of which **one or more** is correct. Select

A	if	**1, 2, and 3**	are correct
B	if	**1 and 3**	are correct
C	if	**2 and 4**	are correct
D	if	**4**	is correct
E	if	**1, 2, 3, and 4**	are correct

247. The list of symptoms specified by *DSM III-R* for the diagnosis of a major depressive episode includes

(1) sleep disturbance
(2) loss of interest or pleasure
(3) significant weight loss
(4) depressed mood

248. Correct statements concerning depression that occurs concomitantly with a medical illness include which of the following?

(1) It may be the result of medication for the organic illness
(2) It has different symptoms than endogenous depression
(3) It may not be related to the organic illness
(4) It typically is unaffected by the course of the organic illness

249. Flight of ideas is a thought process characterized by

(1) rapid speech
(2) abrupt topic changes
(3) punning or plays on words
(4) goal-directed thought

250. The *DSM III-R* criteria for a major depressive episode specify that delusions or hallucinations

(1) must be mood incongruent
(2) must not be present as a major symptom
(3) must be primarily associated with guilt feelings
(4) must not have been present for 2 weeks or more in the absence of prominent mood symptoms

251. A person presents with an acute psychosis that includes symptoms and signs of both mania and schizophrenia. The diagnosis is more likely to be bipolar affective disorder if the person has a family history of

(1) affective disorder
(2) psychiatric illness responsive to lithium
(3) alcoholism
(4) organic brain syndrome

252. Contraindications to the use of ECT include which of the following disorders?

(1) Peptic ulcer
(2) Aortic aneurysm
(3) Glaucoma
(4) Brain tumor

SUMMARY OF DIRECTIONS

A	B	C	D	E
1,2,3 only	1,3 only	2,4 only	4 only	All are correct

253. According to *DSM III-R*, the criteria for a diagnosis of cyclothymia include

(1) a chronic mood disturbance of at least 2 years' duration
(2) numerous manic episodes and periods of depressed mood
(3) a 2-year period in which the person is never without the required symptoms for more than 2 months
(4) an onset in adolescence

254. Personality disorders frequently associated with dysthymia include

(1) borderline personality disorder
(2) histrionic personality disorder
(3) dependent personality disorder
(4) obsessive personality disorder

255. According to *DSM III-R*, the criteria required for the diagnosis of dysthymia (depressive neurosis) include which of the following?

(1) Depressed mood most of the time for at least 2 years
(2) Symptoms while depressed that can include poor appetite, overeating, and low energy or fatigue
(3) No absence of a depressed mood for more than 2 months during a 2-year period
(4) No evidence of a major depressive episode during the first 2 years of the disturbance

256. Signs and symptoms of mania can include

(1) hyperactivity
(2) decreased sleep
(3) distractibility
(4) irritability

DIRECTIONS: The group of questions below consists of lettered headings followed by a set of numbered items. For each numbered item select the **one** lettered heading with which it is **most** closely associated. Each lettered heading may be used **once, more than once, or not at all.**

Questions 257–260

Each statement listed below refers to an etiologic theory of depression. Select the name most closely associated with each statement.

(A) Kraepelin
(B) Lewinsohn
(C) Abraham
(D) Beck
(E) Seligman

257. In contrast to the usual mourner's grief over the lost person, the depressed person is concerned with loss and guilt resulting from unconscious hostility toward the lost person

258. Depression results from specific cognitive distortions present in depression-prone people

259. Depression relates to "learned helplessness"

260. The depressed person lacks social skills, and a decrease in pleasant events or an increase in unpleasant events leads to dysphoria and self-blame, which are then reinforced by the environment

DIRECTIONS: The group of questions below consists of four lettered headings followed by a set of numbered items. For each numbered item select

A	if the item is associated with	(A) **only**
B	if the item is associated with	(B) **only**
C	if the item is associated with	**both** (A) and (B)
D	if the item is associated with	**neither** (A) nor (B)

Each lettered heading may be used **once, more than once, or not at all.**

Questions 261–265

(A) Melancholic major depression
(B) Manic episode
(C) Both
(D) Neither

261. Irritability

262. Predominant sadness, hopelessness

263. Grandiose ideas

264. History of schizophrenia

265. Decreased sexual drive

Mood Disorders

Answers

230. The answer is B. *(Stoudemire, p 625.)* A great many studies have been done to determine the side effects of oral contraceptives, and the results are somewhat inconsistent. Most, however, suggest that the majority of women have no significant side effects. Many, but not all, studies report an increased incidence of depression.

231. The answer is D. *(Michels, vol 1, chap 60, pp 10, 11.)* The evidence for a genetic factor in bipolar affective disorders is reasonably sound. The concordance rate for bipolar illness in monozygotic twins averages 75 percent, when various studies are combined. The concordance rate in dizygotic twins and siblings is 20 to 25 percent, which is significantly higher than that found in the general population.

232. The answer is E. *(Michels, vol 2, chap 19, p 13.)* The treatment of a grief reaction is based on the presumption that it is a normal process, usually of brief duration. Any situation that provides grieving people a chance to express their feelings can be quite supportive. This function most often is provided by family or friends. Antidepressants or long-term psychotherapy is not indicated unless grieving is prolonged or a more severe depression develops.

233. The answer is D. *(Stoudemire, p 579.)* Carcinoma of the pancreas has long been associated with the occurrence of emotional disorder, and the most commonly described symptoms are depression and an intense sense of dread. The incidence of depression that predates the discovery of the malignancy varies from 10 to 50 percent. The symptoms are often similar to those of a major depressive episode, with or without vegetative signs.

234. The answer is E. *(American Psychiatric Association, ed 3-R. pp 230–233.)* Dysthymia is a chronic depression lasting more than 2 years, usually beginning in late adolescence or early adulthood. Sometimes patients describe being depressed for as long as they can remember. Symptoms fluctuate but are usually not severe. Such patients are commonly concerned with their perceived failures or interpersonal disappointments. The somatic symptoms characteristic of major depression or melancholia are less prominent in dysthymia.

235. The answer is A. *(Michels, vol 1, chap 61, pp 13, 14.)* People with typical unipolar depression ruminate about guilt, suicide, somatic fears, or other depressive themes. Concentration and recent-memory impairment, which at first may suggest an organic brain syndrome, improve with the lifting of depression. Concentration and memory difficulties that are secondary to the depression also may be difficult to distinguish from the side effects of antidepressant medication; thus, these symptoms should be carefully assessed before initiation of pharmacotherapy. Although the content of depressive thinking may be delusional or gruesome, the associations or connections characterizing the thought processes of depressed persons are usually conventional and seldom bizarre.

236. The answer is C. *(Stoudemire, pp 636–638.)* Approximately 50 to 80 percent of new mothers will experience "maternity blues" within the first week after delivery, usually resolving within 2 to 3 weeks. When the symptoms persist beyond the first postpartum month, and especially when the symptoms are particularly severe, a postpartum depression must be considered. It appears to occur in about 10 to 15 percent of new mothers, the symptoms are quite similar to those of major depression, and it is treated in a similar fashion.

237. The answer is A. *(Kaplan, ed 4. p 679.)* The therapeutic effect of ECT depends on the production of a seizure. (In fact, convulsions have a beneficial effect on depression, whether they are induced electrically or with medication.) Subconvulsive electrical stimuli can produce loss of consciousness and memory and may even meet a person's wish for punishment, but these results have no effect on the lifting of depression.

238. The answer is C. *(Talbott, p 404.)* Suicide is an ever present danger in seriously depressed persons. The clinician must constantly be on the alert for the signs and symptoms of potential suicide, even in patients who appear to be responding to treatment. It is estimated that approximately 15 percent of seriously depressed persons will eventually kill themselves.

239. The answer is E. *(Talbott, pp 1021–1033.)* Suicide is the ninth leading cause of death in the United States and is most often preventable. The vast majority of victims suffer from psychiatric illness, and the most common is mood disorder. Mood disorder has been identified in 40 to 80 percent of a consecutive series of suicides, and alcoholism in 20 to 30 percent. Males tend to be more successful than females in their attempts, and there is a clear familial association. It is estimated that up to 80 percent of suicide victims have communicated their intent to others, and thus such communications must be taken very seriously.

240. The answer is B. *(American Psychiatric Association, ed 3-R. p 225. Kaplan, ed 4. pp 248, 249.)* The bipolar-unipolar distinction is made entirely on the basis of mania. A current manic episode or a history of mania establishes the diagnosis of bipolar disorder. The bipolar category is classified as depressed, manic or mixed depending on the clinical presentation. The term *unipolar* is not part of official classification, but is used by some clinicians for recurrent major depression.

241. The answer is A. *(American Psychiatric Association, ed 3-R. p 224.)* In the melancholic type of major depression, the patient typically complains of feeling worse in the morning. This is often associated with early morning awakening. As the day progresses, some patients will report a reduction in their feelings of depression.

242. The answer is D. *(Talbott, p 142. Whybrow, pp 81–92.)* Heinz Kohut, originally a classical analyst, ultimately developed a theory of psychopathology emphasizing developmental deficit, as opposed to fixation and regression related to conflict regarding sexual and aggressive drives. He believed that the most important line of development related to the self, and especially to self-esteem and self-cohesion. The development of a cohesive self requires phase-appropriate empathy, in the form of mirroring and idealization from important objects ("selfobjects").

243. The answer is C. *(American Psychiatric Association, ed 3-R. p 220. Michels, vol 2, chap 100, pp 4, 5.)* Persons having a major depressive episode with psychotic features meet diagnostic criteria for depression and have a disturbance of reality-testing manifested by delusions, hallucinations, or severe depressive stupor. Delusional thinking is most frequent and is characterized most commonly by delusions of guilt or sinfulness. Paranoid delusions also are relatively common in this group; however, they usually are associated with guilt-ridden beliefs. Somatic delusions and nihilistic delusions also may occur.

244. The answer is B. *(American Psychiatric Association, ed 3-R. p 229.)* Patients with dysthymia may develop a major depression. When they do, this is sometimes referred to as *double depression*. Such patients are at greater risk for having a recurrence of a major depressive episode than are those patients who have only major depression.

245. The answer is B. *(American Psychiatric Association, ed 3-R. pp 228–230.)* All the statements specify diagnostic criteria for recurrent major depression, except for the statement regarding a symptom-free period. The criteria in *DSM III-R* state that there must be a period of at least 2 months between major depressive episodes, during which the patient returns to more or less usual functioning. It is estimated that about 50 percent of persons who initially have a single episode will eventually have another. People with recurrent major depression are also at greater risk for developing bipolar disorder than are those with a single episode.

246. The answer is B. *(American Psychiatric Association, ed 3-R. pp 225–226.)* Bipolar disorder occurs in about 0.4 to 1.2 percent of the adult population and is equally common in males and females. In the typical case, the initial episode is manic rather than depressed. The periods of disturbance in this disorder tend to be more frequent than the episodes of depression in recurrent major depression. The time interval between episodes in bipolar disorder are variable, but the so-called rapid cyclers tend to have a more chronic course.

247. The answer is E (all). *(American Psychiatric Association, ed 3-R. pp 222–223.)* All the named symptoms are among those for which *DSM III-R* requires that at least five be present for the diagnosis of major depressive episode. Other specified symptoms include psychomotor agitation or retardation, fatigue or loss of energy, feelings of worthlessness or excessive/inappropriate guilt, diminished ability to think or concentrate, and recurrent thoughts of death or suicide. The criteria specify, however, that at least one of the symptoms must be either depressed mood or loss of interest/pleasure. The depressed mood should be present most of the day, nearly every day; and the loss of interest or pleasure should be in most activities and most of the time. In both instances these criteria can be met by either the subjective account of the patient or by the observations of others.

248. The answer is B (1, 3). *(Michels, vol 2, chap 99, pp 1–7.)* Although depression can occur as the first manifestation of organic illness, the discovery of a medical illness does not necessarily explain the genesis of a depression. Depression that is secondary to medical illness is often indistinguishable on the basis of symptoms from primary depression. Depression also may be the result of the treatment of an organic illness rather than a result of the illness itself. Whatever its cause, once depression has begun it may well be aggravated or prolonged by a medical illness.

249. The answer is A (1, 2, 3). *(American Psychiatric Association, ed 3-R. p 215.)* A primary sign of mania, flight of ideas is a train of thoughts that is rapid and pressured. Although manic persons displaying flight of ideas usually lose sight of the original goal or point of their thoughts, the actual associations from one thought to the next are usually understandable and often are clever or humorous. In contrast, the thought associations of schizophrenic persons are more frequently bizarre and incomprehensible. In severe manic psychosis, associations may also become incomprehensible and speech disorganized.

250. The answer is D (4). *(American Psychiatric Association, ed 3-R. p 223.)* Delusions and hallucinations may be associated with the diagnosis of a major depressive episode, but they are not required for the diagnosis. Often, but not always, they are associated with feelings of worthlessness or inappropriate or excessive guilt. Delusions or hallucinations must not have been present for more than 2 weeks prior to the development of mood symptoms, or after the mood symptoms have remitted. This helps to differentiate major depression from other psychoses that may have associated mood symptoms.

251. The answer is A (1, 2, 3). *(Kaplan, ed 4. pp 248, 249.)* It is not uncommon for people with an acute psychosis to have symptoms and signs of both mania and schizophrenia. In the past, American psychiatrists tended to diagnose such patients as schizophrenic or schizoaffective, presuming schizophrenia to be the basic disorder. The effectiveness of lithium therapy for the treatment of bipolar illness makes the distinction between affective and schizophrenic disease a crucial therapeutic task. Currently, it is suggested that when the acute symptomatic picture is mixed, a family history of affective disorder, alcoholism or psychiatric illness treated successfully by lithium therapy favors the diagnosis of bipolar illness.

252. The answer is D (4). *(Kaplan, ed 4. pp 682, 683.)* The only absolute contraindication to the use of ECT is the presence of a brain tumor. During therapy, intracerebral pressure rises, posing a significant risk to patients with brain tumors. ECT does not increase the risk of hemorrhage in such medical conditions as peptic ulcer and aortic aneurysm; also, because intraocular pressure actually drops during a convulsion, glaucoma is not adversely affected. The effect of pretreatment medications on a patient's medical status must be considered before initiation of ECT.

253. The answer is B (1, 3). *(American Psychiatric Association, ed 3-R. pp 226–228.)* The essential feature of cyclothymia is a chronic mood disturbance of at least 2 years' duration (1 year for children and adolescents), during which there are numerous hypomanic episodes and periods of depressed mood or loss of interest or pleasure. However, the symptoms must not be of sufficient severity or duration to meet the criteria for major depressive or manic episodes. The affected person must never be without the required symptoms for more than 2 months in a 2-year period (1 year for children and adolescents). The diagnosis cannot be made if the disturbance is superimposed on another chronic psychotic disorder, such as schizophrenia, or maintained by an organic factor or substance abuse. Some investigators believe that this is a mild form of bipolar disorder. While the age of onset is usually in adolescence or early adulthood, it can occur either earlier or later. A particular age of onset is not one of the diagnostic requirements.

254. The answer is A (1, 2, 3). *(American Psychiatric Association, ed 3-R. p 232.)* People with dysthymia often display a concurrent personality disorder. The personality traits or disorders most commonly associated with dysthymia are borderline, histrionic, narcissistic, avoidant, and dependent types. Obsessive traits are more characteristic of people with melancholia.

255. The answer is E (all). *(American Psychiatric Association, ed 3-R. pp 230–233.)* All the factors listed are part of the *DSM III-R* criteria for a diagnosis of dysthymia. Of the specific symptoms listed in choice 2, only two need to be present during the period of depression. The list also includes insomnia or hypersomnia, low self-esteem, poor concentration, difficulty in making decisions, and feelings of hopelessness. In children and adolescents the requirement is modified such that the depressed mood must not be absent for more than 2 months during a 1-year period. The patient may still have this diagnosis if there was a previous major depressive episode more than 2 years before the disturbance, as long as there was a full remission such that there were no signs or symptoms for at least 6 months. If a major depression develops after a 2-year period of dysthymia, both diagnoses are given. Additional requirements for this diagnosis include an absence of any previous manic or hypomanic episodes and that the disturbance not be superimposed on a chronic psychotic disorder. Also, it cannot be initiated or maintained by an organic factor, for example the prolonged administration of an antihypertensive medication.

256. The answer is E (all). *(American Psychiatric Association, ed 3-R. pp 214–218.)* Primary signs of mania include euphoria or irritable mood. Manic persons frequently are grandiose and easily distracted. They often describe their own energy level as boundless, have increased activity, need less sleep, dress in a bizarre or flamboyant manner, and engage in spending sprees.

257–260. The answers are: 257-C, 258-D, 259-E, 260-B. *(Talbott, pp 405, 424–427.)* Kraepelin was a pioneer in the classification of psychiatric disorders early in this century. He emphasized the longitudinal history and pattern of symptoms. He differentiated what he called manic-depressive illness (major depression, bipolar disorder, and some patients with dysthymia) from dementia praecox (schizophrenia). He noted that the former had an episodic and relatively benign course, while the latter was often chronic and deteriorating.

Abraham (1911) was an early psychoanalytic theorist who noted that unlike the usual mourner who grieves, the depressed person is preoccupied with guilt, loss, and inadequacy that are based on unconscious hostility toward the lost person. Freud (1917) expanded on these theories to note that, unlike the usual mourner, the depressed person is unable to resolve these ambivalent feelings. The anger toward the lost person is turned inward, resulting in dysphoria, guilt, and loss of self-esteem.

Lewinsohn (1974) proposed that the person who is likely to become depressed is one who lacks social skills. A subsequent decrease in response-contingent positive reinforcement (a decrease in pleasant events or an increase in unpleasant events) then leads to dysphoria and self-blame. Once the depression begins, the secondary gain (positive reinforcement from sympathy, attention, and so on) escalates the condition to the level of clinical depression.

Aaron Beck (1972) proposed a cognitive-behavioral model of depression. Depression-prone people have specific cognitive distortions (''depressogenic schemata'') derived from early experience. These disturbed cognitions result in unrealistically negative views of self, world, and future.

Seligman proposed that experiences with uncontrollable events lead to cognitive and emotional deficits that result in a state of ''learned-helplessness.'' The resultant expectations and conclusions about self and life events can result in depression.

261–265. The answers are: 261-C, 262-A, 263-B, 264-D, 265-A. *(American Psychiatric Association, ed 3-R. pp 214–224.)* Melancholic depression and mania are both major affective disorders. Melancholia includes clinical manifestations such as irritability, severe sadness, anhedonia, crying, hopelessness, helplessness, impaired memory, pessimism, delusions of inadequacy or punishment, suicidal thoughts, social withdrawal, and decreased sex drive. It is not associated with a history of schizophrenia.

Mania, or the manic phase of bipolar affective disorder, is characterized by a euphoric, expansive mood state. Like melancholia, irritability is common, as is poor concentration. These patients are easily distractible, have flight of ideas, and express grandiose thoughts. They are uninhibited and show an increased sex drive. The mood is typically labile. Although sometimes misdiagnosed as schizophrenia, there is no relationship.

Anxiety, Somatoform, and Dissociative Disorders

DIRECTIONS: Each question below contains five suggested responses. Select the **one best** response to each question.

266. Patients with panic disorder are usually

(A) male
(B) hospitalized
(C) older than 40
(D) severely incapacitated
(E) seen by medical physicians

267. All the following statements about agoraphobia are true EXCEPT

(A) it is more common in females
(B) it is rarely accompanied by panic disorder
(C) it may result in the patient being totally housebound
(D) it is frequently associated with a fear of being alone
(E) it often has an onset between 20 and 30 years of age

268. All the following are true statements about multiple personality disorder EXCEPT

(A) the onset is usually in childhood
(B) there is often a history of childhood abuse
(C) the disorder is more common in females
(D) only one personality recurrently takes full control of the person's behavior
(E) the transition from one personality to another is usually sudden

269. All the following statements about generalized anxiety disorder are true EXCEPT

(A) there is persistent anxiety lasting for at least 1 month
(B) the disorder is equally common in females and males
(C) the onset is usually in young adulthood
(D) symptoms include vigilance and scanning
(E) mild depressive symptoms are common

270. Which of the following statements describes conversion disorder?

(A) It is much more frequently associated with major sensorimotor disturbances today than 50 years ago
(B) Charcot believed it was caused by hereditary degeneration of the central nervous system
(C) It is associated exclusively with histrionic personality
(D) Its somatic manifestations are mediated predominantly by the autonomic nervous system
(E) It does little to relieve anxiety

271. Conversion disorder can produce all the following physical disturbances EXCEPT

(A) rhythmic tremors
(B) tongue biting
(C) astasia-abasia
(D) proximal paresis
(E) "gun barrel" vision

DIRECTIONS: Each question below contains four suggested responses of which **one or more** is correct. Select

A	if	**1, 2, and 3**	are correct
B	if	**1 and 3**	are correct
C	if	**2 and 4**	are correct
D	if	**4**	is correct
E	if	**1, 2, 3, and 4**	are correct

272. Panic disorder is often associated with fear of

(1) dying
(2) "going crazy"
(3) being in crowds
(4) heights

273. As a consequence of panic disorder, the patient may develop

(1) generalized anxiety
(2) secondary depression
(3) agoraphobia
(4) psychosis

274. Which of the following can cause symptoms similar to those found in panic disorder?

(1) Pheochromocytoma
(2) Hypoglycemia
(3) Withdrawal from barbiturates
(4) Intoxication with caffeine

275. The locus ceruleus theory for the etiology of panic attacks is supported by the observation that

(1) yohimbine provokes anxiety
(2) electrical stimulation of the locus ceruleus produces anxiety
(3) tricyclic antidepressants may block panic attacks
(4) sodium lactate provokes anxiety in patients without panic disorder

276. During a panic attack, patients commonly experience

(1) shortness of breath
(2) palpitations
(3) dizziness
(4) numbness and tingling

277. Drugs that are clearly effective for prevention of panic attacks include

(1) imipramine
(2) alprazolam
(3) phenelzine
(4) diazepam

278. Alcoholic amnestic disorder is distinguished from psychogenic amnesia by which of the following statements?

(1) Short-term, but not immediate, memory is impaired
(2) There is lack of awareness of impairment of memory
(3) Confabulation is common
(4) Blunted affect is common

279. While the differentiation of anxiety from depression is often difficult, generally patients with generalized anxiety disorder

(1) do not demonstrate the full range of vegetative symptoms seen in depression
(2) do not respond to treatment with tricyclic antidepressants
(3) do not show the diurnal mood fluctuation common to depression
(4) experience dysphoria first, followed by anxiety symptoms

280. Somatization disorder is characterized by

(1) onset in old age
(2) frequent gastrointestinal symptoms
(3) predominance in males
(4) frequent symptoms in organs of special sense

281. Characteristic features of panic disorder include

(1) episodic, recurrent course
(2) signs reminiscent of myocardial infarction or hyperthyroidism
(3) anticipatory helplessness
(4) occurrence during severe stress

282. Agoraphobia can be described by which of the following statements?

(1) Women are affected twice as often as men
(2) Onset is quite unlikely after 40 years of age
(3) Affected persons usually come from close-knit families
(4) Onset is unusual in childhood

283. Nearly everyone has experienced brief episodes of obsessive thinking or compulsive behavior. Features of obsessive compulsive disorder include

(1) onset typically by 15 years of age
(2) equal incidence in men and women
(3) quest for treatment earlier than associated with other neurotic disorders
(4) realization by affected persons that the symptoms are manifestations of a mental disorder

284. Respiratory discomfort associated with acute anxiety attacks can lead to hyperventilation. If continued long enough, hyperventilation can result in

(1) respiratory acidosis
(2) carpopedal spasm
(3) peripheral vasodilation
(4) paresthesia

SUMMARY OF DIRECTIONS

A	B	C	D	E
1,2,3	1,3	2,4	4	All are
only	only	only	only	correct

285. Correct statements about phobias include which of the following?

(1) Agoraphobia is the most common phobic disorder

(2) A cardinal feature of phobias is avoidant behavior stemming from an irrational fear

(3) Phobic anxiety may be compounded by unpleasant depersonalization feelings

(4) The psychological origin of the phobic symptoms is usually quite apparent

DIRECTIONS: Each group of questions below consists of lettered headings followed by a set of numbered items. For each numbered item select the **one** lettered heading with which it is **most** closely associated. Each lettered heading may be used **once, more than once, or not at all.**

Questions 286–288

Match the following.

(A) Agoraphobia
(B) Social Phobia
(C) Simple Phobia
(D) Both simple and social phobia
(E) None of the above

286. Generally elicited by a circumscribed stimulus

287. Characterized by marked fear and avoidance of being alone or in public places, which leads to increased limitations on normal activity

288. Characterized by persistent, irrational fear of humiliation or embarrassment

Questions 289–293

Match the following.

(A) Somatization disorder
(B) Obsessive compulsive disorder
(C) Psychogenic fugue
(D) Body dysmorphic disorder
(E) Posttraumatic stress disorder

289. After watching her house burn down, a 32-year-old woman has recurrent dreams about the event

290. A 20-year-old college student is very upset because his nose looks crooked, though to others it appears normal

291. A nun is found in a distant city, working in a cabaret, and unable to remember her previous life

292. A 35-year-old mother is anxious and upset by her inability to stop persistent impulses to stab her newborn child

293. A college student has a 3-year history of episodes of amnesia and blindness, as well as multiple chest and gastrointestinal symptoms, for which no organic cause can be discovered

Anxiety, Somatoform, and Dissociative Disorders

Answers

266. The answer is E. *(American Psychiatric Association, ed 3-R. pp 235–239.)* Panic disorder most often begins in young adulthood and when associated with agoraphobia it occurs more commonly in females. Patients with panic disorder may develop avoidance behavior so that their activity becomes constricted, but they are usually not severely incapacitated. They are able to care for themselves and usually are not hospitalized. Because the somatic complaints they experience may mimic other medical illnesses and because the patient may not view the problem as "psychological," these patients frequently seek help from medical physicians.

267. The answer is B. *(American Psychiatric Association, ed 3-R. pp 240–241.)* Panic disorder with agoraphobia is much more common than panic disorder without agoraphobia. However, occasionally patients will present with agoraphobia without a history or presence of panic disorder. In this condition the patient experiences the same fears of being in situations from which escape would be difficult, or in which help might not be available in the event that symptoms should develop. Commonly feared symptoms include becoming dizzy, loss of bladder or bowel control, and vomiting. It is unclear as to whether agoraphobia is always a variant of panic disorder.

268. The answer is D. *(American Psychiatric Association, ed 3-R. pp 269–270.)* In adults, the number of personalities in any one case of multiple personality disorder varies from two to over one hundred. Approximately half of recently reported cases have ten personalities or less. At least two of the personalities, at some time and recurrently, take full control of the person's behavior. The disorder commonly has its onset in childhood, though often it is not diagnosed until much later in life. Studies of patients with this disorder consistently reveal a high percentage who have been subjected to sexual or physical abuse in childhood.

269. The answer is A. *(American Psychiatric Association, ed 3-R. pp 251–253.)* According to the criteria of *DSM III-R*, for a diagnosis of generalized anxiety disorder there must be symptoms of unrealistic or excessive anxiety about two or more life circumstances for 6 months or longer. The spectrum of symptoms includes many signs of motor tension, autonomic hyperactivity, vigilance, and scanning. The onset is most commonly in young adulthood, the course is often chronic, and the disorder occurs with equal frequency in males and females. Often there are mild depressive symptoms, and the disorder sometimes seems to follow a major depressive episode.

270. The answer is B. *(Kaplan, ed 4. p 342.)* Traditionally, conversion disorder (conversion "hysteria") is distinguished from psychophysiological disorders in that its manifestations are mediated by the voluntary nervous system. Charcot, who helped pioneer the systematic study of conversion hysteria, believed the disorder was caused by a hereditary degeneration of the central nervous system. Current opinion is that the conversion symptom serves a psychodynamic function: namely, to relieve anxiety. Although classic conversion reactions—paralysis, convulsions, anesthesia, and other major sensorimotor symptoms—are probably seen less often now than 50 years ago, the overall incidence of conversion disorder may not necessarily have declined. A variety of personality types have been associated with conversion disorder.

271. The answer is B. *(Kaplan, ed 4. pp 344–347.)* Physical manifestations of conversion disorder can affect all parts of the body. Persons who have conversion disorder can have rhythmic tremors of their extremities. Although they may have seizures marked by bizarre disorganized movements, even opisthotonos, affected persons rarely injure themselves; tongue biting, bruising, and contusions are quite unlikely to occur during the seizure episode. Astasia-abasia (grossly irregular gait), proximal paresis (not the distal weakness commonly associated with central nervous system disorders), and "gun barrel" vision (uniform constriction of visual fields) also are displayed by people who have conversion disorder.

272. The answer is A (1, 2, 3). *(American Psychiatric Association, ed 3-R. pp 235–241.)* During panic attacks the fear of losing one's mind or "going crazy" is common. Agoraphobia is a consequence of frequent panic attacks and is characterized by fears of being alone or in crowded public places. It is hypothesized that the affected person fears places or situations where he or she will be unable to flee or get help should a panic attack occur. The fear of heights is an example of a simple phobia and differs from panic disorder in that panic attacks do not occur spontaneously but only when the patient is exposed to the fearful situation.

273. The answer is A (1, 2, 3). *(American Psychiatric Association, ed 3-R. pp 235–237. Michels, vol 1, chap 33, p 4.)* As a consequence of panic disorder, patients develop anticipatory anxiety (or generalized anxiety) apparently because they are fearful of the next anxiety attack. Frequently it is difficult for patients later to recall whether the generalized anxiety or the panic attack began first. Agoraphobia, the fear of open or crowded places, may develop as a consequence of panic attacks. Similarly, depression is not uncommon in such patients. Psychosis, however, is not associated with this disorder, even though the fear of losing one's mind, or "going crazy," is common.

274. The answer is E (all). *(American Psychiatric Association, ed 3-R. p 237.)* The differential diagnosis of panic disorder includes several physical conditions. These include disorders such as pheochromocytoma, hyperthyroidism, and hypoglycemia. Also, withdrawal from substances such as barbiturates, and intoxication with substances such as caffeine and amphetamine, can induce panic attacks.

275. The answer is A (1, 2, 3). *(Talbott, p 448.)* The locus ceruleus, located in the pons, is involved in a prominent hypothesis for the etiology of panic attacks. The hypothesis is supported by the observation that electrical stimulation of this area, or its stimulation by drugs such as yohimbine, is associated with an anxiety response. Drugs capable of blocking panic attacks, such as the tricyclic antidepressants, have been shown to curtail locus ceruleus firing. Infusions of sodium lactate induce anxiety in patients with panic disorder, but less frequently or not at all in normal controls.

276. The answer is E (all). *(American Psychiatric Association, ed 3-R. pp 235–239. Michels, vol 1, chap 32, pp 2–4.)* During a panic attack the patient experiences the sudden onset of apprehension or fears something dreadful is about to happen. These fears are associated with a variety of physical symptoms of somatic anxiety. These symptoms commonly include shortness of breath, palpitations, chest pain, choking sensations, dizziness, paresthesias, hot and cold flashes, sweating, and shaking. The patient may seek medical treatment, thinking the episode is a "heart attack" or some other medical problem.

277. The answer is A (1, 2, 3). *(Michels, vol 1, chap 32, pp 11–12.)* Imipramine, a tricyclic antidepressant, and phenelzine, a monoamine oxidase inhibitor, are both more effective than placebo for treatment of panic disorder. Some investigators think phenelzine is the more effective of the two. Recent studies have shown alprazolam to be very effective as well. The benzodiazepines in general are of some value for treating symptoms of anxiety, once present, but are less useful for preventing panic attacks.

278. The answer is E (all). *(American Psychiatric Association, ed 3-R. pp 274–275.)* In psychogenic amnesia there is a sudden inability to recall important personal information. During such an amnestic period the patient may exhibit perplexity, disorientation, and purposeless wandering. When the amnesia is for the past, the patient is usually aware of the disturbance of recall. In alcoholic amnestic disorder, events can be recalled immediately after they occur, but not after a few minutes. This is not seen in psychogenic amnesia. Also, the patient commonly displays blunted affect, confabulation, and a lack of awareness of the short-term memory impairment.

279. The answer is B (1, 3). *(Talbott, pp 453–454.)* The differentiation of anxiety from depression can be very difficult because anxious patients can be depressed and depressed patients can be quite anxious. Patients with generalized anxiety disorder or panic disorder generally do not show the full range of vegetative symptoms seen in a depressive episode. They may have difficulty falling asleep, but usually do not show early morning awakening, loss of appetite, loss of the ability to concentrate, or diurnal mood fluctuation. Anxious patients also do not show an equivalent loss of the capacity to enjoy things. Also, they generally give a history of having anxiety symptoms first, followed by the gradual development of dysphoric symptoms. Depressed patients usually give a history of feeling dysphoria first, with anxiety symptoms coming later. Tricyclic antidepressants are commonly used in the treatment of both panic disorder and depression.

280. The answer is C (2, 4). *(Michels, vol 1, chap 35, pp 1–19.)* People with somatization disorder are frequently sickly as children and criteria specify onset before age 30. Gastrointestinal symptoms (lump in throat, vomiting, nausea, and diarrhea) and conversion symptoms in organs of special sense (blindness and aphoria) occur at least three times more frequently than in control patients. In addition, symptoms in sex organs and paralysis or pain in extremities may be found. The disorder is much more common in women.

281. The answer is A (1, 2, 3). *(Kaplan, ed 4. p 316.)* Panic disorder is a recurrent disorder characterized by acute panic anxiety and feelings of helplessness and fear preceding the panic attack. Affected persons often do remarkably well during times of severe life stress, and exertion is not known to bring about an attack. Symptoms and signs can include tremor, sweating, hyperreflexia, tachycardia, dyspnea, palpitations, and hyperventilation. As a consequence, the differential diagnosis of patients presenting with an apparent panic attack should include other disorders—such as angina, myocardial infarction, hyperthyroidism, and pheochromocytoma—also associated with these common constitutional symptoms.

282. The answer is E (all). *(Kaplan, ed 4. pp 323–324.)* Twice as many women as men suffer from agoraphobia (dread of public encounters). Typically present in the histories of affected persons is a close-knit family. Onset of agoraphobic disorders usually occurs between 20 and 40 years of age; children do not experience this type of phobia.

283. The answer is E (all). *(Kaplan, ed 4. pp 328–332.)* Two-thirds of persons with obsessive compulsive disorder describe symptoms by 15 years of age, and 10 to 15 percent by 10 years of age. It is uncommon for symptoms to appear first after 30 years of age. Affected persons often seek help for their disabling disorder in early adulthood, or about 10 years sooner than persons with other neurotic disorders. People with obsessive compulsive disorder are keenly aware of and uncomfortable with their symptoms, viewed by them as "foreign bodies" in their psychic and behavioral lives.

284. The answer is C (2, 4). *(Kaplan, ed 4. pp 511–512.)* Persons experiencing an acute anxiety attack commonly complain of respiratory discomfort. A feeling of air hunger can cause them to pant and hyperventilate. Prolonged hyperventilation can lower the P_{CO2} and produce respiratory alkalosis. Peripheral vasoconstriction can cause paresthesia of the extremities and carpopedal spasm. Development of these symptoms may fuel the anxiety and increase the feeling of panic.

285. The answer is A (1, 2, 3). *(Kaplan, ed 4. pp 151, 152, 179.)* Phobias usually involve an inexplicable fear, sometimes approaching panic. Affected persons characteristically avoid the phobic situation or object. Associated symptoms of phobia can include psychophysiological signs of panic—dizziness, air hunger, flushing, and palpitations. Depersonalization, which is the sensation of feeling separated from portions of or all of one's own body, also can occur. The origins of any given phobia are obscure at the outset and can be uncovered only by a period of psychotherapy. Agoraphobia, a fear of public places or of leaving home, constitutes 60 percent of all phobias. Phobias affect less than 1 percent of the general population.

286–288. The answers are: 286-D, 287-A, 288-B. *(American Psychiatric Association, ed 3-R. pp 241–245. Michels, vol 1, chap 33, pp 6–7.)* Phobic disorders, a subclassification of anxiety disorders, include agoraphobia and simple and social phobias. They are all characterized by overwhelming, persistent, and irrational fears that result in the overpowering need to avoid the object or situation generating the dread. Agoraphobia is the marked fear and avoidance of being alone or in public places where rapid exit would be difficult. As the phobia progresses, avoidance of the stimulus dominates the person's life. Social phobia is characterized by avoidance of situations in which one is exposed to scrutiny by others and a fear of being humiliated or embarrassed by one's actions. Simple phobias are triggered by objects—often animals or insects—heights, or closed spaces. A large variety of objects are associated with simple phobias. Both social and simple phobias generally involve a circumscribed stimulus that elicits the phobic response.

289–293. The answers are: 289-E, 290-D, 291-C, 292-B, 293-A. *(American Psychiatric Association, ed 3-R. pp 245–251, 255–256, 261–264, 272–273).* One of the characteristic features of posttraumatic stress disorder is the occurrence of repeated dreams or recollections of the major stress event. The disturbance must persist for more than 1 month for the diagnosis to be made.

In body dysmorphic disorder, a person of normal appearance is preoccupied with some imagined insignificant physical anomaly. The belief is not of delusional intensity, for if it were it would be diagnosed as a delusional disorder. The diagnosis also specifically excludes both anorexia nervosa, wherein thin patients see themselves as obese, and transexualism.

In psychogenic fugue, the predominant disturbance is sudden, unexpected travel, with inability to recall one's past. There is a partial or complete assumption of a new identity, often one that is more uninhibited.

Patients with obsessive compulsive disorder have persistent thoughts, impulses, or compulsions that are very stressful and that they are unable to stop by act of will. These are experienced as intrusive, senseless products of one's own mind. They are the source of much distress and interference.

In somatization disorder, a patient without evidence of organic pathology has at least 13 physical symptoms from a list that includes gastrointestinal, cardiopulmonary, sexual, conversion or pseudoneurologic, and pain symptoms. The condition begins before age 30 and usually has a chronic though fluctuating course. It is most commonly diagnosed in females.

Personality Disorders, Human Sexuality, and Miscellaneous Syndromes

DIRECTIONS: Each question below contains five suggested responses. Select the **one best** response to each question.

294. All the following are associated with narcissistic personality disorder EXCEPT

(A) intense empathy
(B) fantasies of glory
(C) entitlement
(D) exploitative behavior
(E) grandiose self-importance

295. The differential diagnosis of obsessive compulsive personality disorder includes all the following conditions EXCEPT

(A) depression
(B) anxiety disorders
(C) phobias
(D) schizophrenia
(E) impulse disorders

296. All the following statements concerning persons with avoidant personality disorder are true EXCEPT

(A) they usually appear calm during psychiatric interviews
(B) they very much want affection and are eager to please
(C) they require uncritical acceptance before entering into a relationship
(D) in their work, they usually are on the periphery of responsibility
(E) they are hypersensitive to rejection and misinterpret social interactions

297. The most common finding in patients with factitious disorder is

(A) an associated major mental disorder
(B) an aggressive, assertive personality style
(C) frequent signings out of hospital
(D) self-administered injections or self-medication
(E) lack of medical training

298. Phobias would be LEAST likely to occur in conjunction with or as manifestations of which of the following disorders?

(A) Schizophrenia
(B) Depersonalization states
(C) Sociopathy
(D) Obsessive states
(E) Anorexia nervosa

299. The diagnosis of adjustment disorder is limited to those patients who have a

(A) specific psychiatric disorder exacerbated by stress
(B) maladaptive reaction to a single, overwhelming life stress
(C) maladaptive reaction that ceases promptly after the precipitating stress has passed
(D) maladaptive dysfunctional reaction markedly out of proportion to the severity of the precipitating stress
(E) reactive disturbance of emotion but no disturbance of conduct

300. Children who go on to develop antisocial personality disorder in adulthood would be LEAST likely to

(A) engage in thievery
(B) attempt suicide
(C) be truant
(D) stay out late
(E) run away

301. All the following statements describe Ganser's syndrome EXCEPT that

(A) it may be a subtype of malingering
(B) it was first described in criminals awaiting trial for serious offenses
(C) it can be mistaken for dementia
(D) affected persons' responses are unrelated to questions asked them
(E) it is considered to be a disorder of both thought and speech

302. All the following are characteristics of multiple personality disorder (MPD) EXCEPT that

(A) observers are usually unaware of personality changes
(B) MPD is considered a dissociative disorder in *DSM III-R*
(C) afflicted persons find objects in their possession they cannot account for
(D) hypnosis may facilitate diagnosis
(E) the disorder is frequently not recognized

DIRECTIONS: Each question below contains four suggested responses of which **one or more** is correct. Select

A	if	**1, 2, and 3**	are correct
B	if	**1 and 3**	are correct
C	if	**2 and 4**	are correct
D	if	**4**	is correct
E	if	**1, 2, 3, and 4**	are correct

303. Advantages of multidimensional self-rated instruments used to assess personality include which of the following?

(1) They provide useful supplementary information
(2) They assist in making diagnostic and treatment decisions
(3) They are relatively cost-effective
(4) They diminish the possibility of inter-rater bias

304. Schizoid personality disorder is differentiated from schizotypal personality disorder by

(1) an absence of close relationships and friends
(2) constricted affect
(3) avoidance of social situations
(4) an absence of oddities of behavior, perception, and speech

305. Empirically based psychometric instruments used to assess personality disorders include which of the following?

(1) Minnesota multiphasic personality inventory (MMPI)
(2) Thematic apperception test (TAT)
(3) Clinical analysis questionnaire (CAQ)
(4) Profile of mood state (POMS)

306. The circumplex model is useful in making the diagnosis of which of the following conditions?

(1) Schizophrenia
(2) Anxiety disorders
(3) Somatoform disorders
(4) Personality disorders

307. Medical complications commonly found in bulimia nervosa include

(1) hypokalemic alkalosis
(2) parotid gland enlargement
(3) cardiac arrhythmias or failure
(4) gastric dilatation

308. True statements concerning personality disorders include that

(1) personality disorders are relatively superficial and respond well to therapy
(2) personality disorders cause impairment in adaptive functioning or subjective distress
(3) persons with personality disorders can have periods of remission up to a year
(4) personality disorders are evident by adolescence or earlier

309. People who have dependent personality disorder are characterized by

(1) a lack of suggestibility
(2) a generally optimistic outlook on life
(3) a subtle sense of self-confidence
(4) an ability to lure others into taking major responsibility for their lives

310. According to the criteria of *DSM III-R*, personality disorders are

(1) coded on axis II
(2) not diagnosed in the presence of major mental illness
(3) recognizable by adolescence or early adult life
(4) not associated with impairment of social/vocational functioning

311. Transsexualism, a gender identity disorder, can be described by which of the following statements?

(1) Most transsexuals deny their anatomical sex
(2) Clinical presentation of male transsexualism can vary considerably
(3) Sex-change operations are deleterious in the long term to transsexuals
(4) The main characteristic of transsexualism is the feeling of being a man or woman in the body of the opposite gender

Questions 312–314

A 17-year-old high-school senior, who is 168 cm (66 in) tall and weighs 31.8 kg (70 lb) is admitted to the hospital. She talks a great deal about fears of "losing control" and becoming fat. She diets rigorously and exercises faithfully; and, though emaciated in appearance, she insists that her cheeks, abdomen, hips, and thighs are too heavy. She is unconcerned that her menstrual periods have ceased. The clinical staff notes that, though busy about the kitchen on her ward, she orders dietary food, spreads it about her plate, and eats little. Her parents are concerned about her weight but are not sure she should be hospitalized.

312. Important symptoms and signs associated with this condition include

(1) striving for thinness
(2) altered body image
(3) amenorrhea
(4) behavioral problems at home

313. Clinical and laboratory examination of the girl described above would be likely to reveal

(1) bradycardia
(2) elevated serum carotene concentration
(3) hypotension and hypothermia
(4) leukopenia

314. The girl described is likely to

(1) ignore concerns about dying
(2) display a strong wish to remain passively dependent
(3) have obsessional traits
(4) have an underlying depression

315. Transvestism (fetishistic cross-dressing) can be described by which of the following statements?

(1) It occurs exclusively in males and usually begins in adolescence
(2) Unlike male transsexuals, male transvestites do not wish to be women
(3) The behavior serves the purpose of promoting sexual arousal and often becomes the only means by which sexual arousal can occur
(4) Male transvestites who wish to pass in public as women have a better prognosis in treatment than men whose behavior is more purely fetishistic

316. Folie à deux can be described by which of the following statements?

(1) It is not always dependent upon close emotional bonds between the participants
(2) It has a good prognosis when it occurs in the geriatric population
(3) Persons with this condition are highly intelligent and live in good economic circumstances
(4) Treatment of the passive partner should include compensation for the loss of the dominant partner

317. Anorexia nervosa is characterized by which of the following?

(1) An intense fear of obesity
(2) Distorted body image—"feeling fat" even when emaciated
(3) Refusal to maintain weight over minimum normal weight
(4) Weight loss of at least 35 percent of original body weight

318. Munchausen's syndrome can be characterized by which of the following statements?

(1) Long-term psychotherapy is the treatment of choice
(2) The disorder, though hard to manage, is relatively easy to recognize
(3) Histrionic and antisocial personality disorders are common diagnoses in affected patients
(4) Affected patients become dependent and ingratiating when hospitalized

319. Capgras' syndrome can be described by which of the following statements?

(1) Affected persons describe other, usually familiar persons as imposters
(2) The disorder is similar to false memories of familiarity, such as déjà vu
(3) Cognitive and perceptual processes are disrupted
(4) The disorder is a form of a neurotic dissociative reaction

320. Characteristics of people who have paranoid personality disorder include

(1) overconcern with hidden motives and special meanings
(2) preoccupation with helping the weak and powerless
(3) extreme reluctance to enter into psychotherapy
(4) predisposition to develop schizophrenia

321. Genetic studies of personality characteristics clearly support which of the following conclusions?

(1) Heredity seems more influential than environment in the development of social introversion
(2) Obsessive compulsive disorder occurs in a high percentage of relatives of affected persons
(3) Histrionic, extroverted persons display lower sedation thresholds than do depressive, introverted people
(4) Adoptees whose adopted parents are schizophrenic but whose biological parents are not have an increased tendency to develop schizotypal personality traits

322. Persons with antisocial personality disorder typically do which of the following?

(1) Convey an impression of intelligence to psychiatric examiners
(2) Explain their behavior away with an appropriate expressing of feeling
(3) "Burn out" (i.e., remit) by mid-adulthood
(4) Respond to a brief course of limit-setting psychotherapy

323. Passive aggressive personality disorder is frequently associated with

(1) obstructionism, stubbornness, and deliberate inefficiency
(2) alcoholism
(3) depression
(4) eventual development of schizophrenia

324. Correct statements concerning disorders of impulse control include which of the following?

(1) Kleptomania and pathological gambling are subtypes of the disorder
(2) Most persons displaying pyromania and "intermittent explosive disorder" are male
(3) Intermittent explosive disorder typically affects teenagers and young adults
(4) The impulsive action is egosyntonic at the time it is performed

325. People who have borderline personality disorder can be described by which of the following statements?

(1) They usually avoid dependence in close relationships
(2) Their reasoning on unstructured psychological tests (e.g., the Rorschach test) is usually normal
(3) They usually respond well to regressive psychotherapy
(4) They characteristically respond to crisis with intense anger

DIRECTIONS: The group of questions below consists of four lettered headings followed by a set of numbered items. For each numbered item select

A	if the item is associated with	(A) **only**
B	if the item is associated with	(B) **only**
C	if the item is associated with	**both** (A) and (B)
D	if the item is associated with	**neither** (A) nor (B)

Each lettered heading may be used **once, more than once, or not at all.**

Questions 326–330

(A) Schizoid personality disorder
(B) Avoidant personality disorder
(C) Both
(D) Neither

326. Hypersensitivity to rejection

327. Few personal attachments

328. Absence of warm, tender feelings for others

329. Eccentricities of speech and behavior common

330. Low self-esteem

Personality Disorders, Human Sexuality, and Miscellaneous Syndromes

Answers

294. The answer is A. *(Talbott, pp 632–633.)* All the listed characteristics are found in narcissistic personality disorder except empathy. Patients with this disorder are notable for their lack of empathy and consideration for the feelings of others. This is associated with a grandiose sense of self-importance, and a sense of entitlement. As a result their relationships tend to be self-centered and shallow.

295. The answer is E. *(Kaplan, ed 4. p 333.)* Obsessive compulsive personality features can be associated with several psychiatric disorders. They can occur in depressive syndromes as well as in phobic states. An increase in obsessional thinking and compulsive behavior may herald a schizophrenic breakdown. Obsessive compulsive people typically are cautious, controlled, and anxious, in contrast to people who have impulse disorders.

296. The answer is A. *(Kaplan, ed 4. pp 377–378.)* Persons with an avoidant personality disorder are anxious, often strikingly so, during psychiatric interviews. They typically are eager to please yet are oversensitive to perceived rejection. Despite low self-esteem and avoidance of risk, these persons desire almost desperately to be in the social and occupational mainstream. Usually, however, their relationships are distorted by their exquisite sensitivity to rejection, and they gravitate toward work roles far from the spotlight. Alliance with a therapist and assertiveness training may be quite helpful to persons who have avoidant personality disorder.

297. The answer is D. *(Michels, vol 1, chap 35, pp 16–19.)* Patients with factitious disorders are often medical professionals or people closely associated with and knowledgeable about hospitals. Self-administered injections or ingestions of medication or foreign material (e.g., insulin, contaminants producing infection, or unacknowledged misuse of prescribed medication) are typical modes of simulating illness. These people are often passive and immature and create much controversy and anxiety in personnel who are treating them. When these patients are confronted with the diagnosis of factitious disorder, their abnormal behavior is best interpreted to them as their cry for help. Suicide attempts and signing out of hospitals are infrequent even after confrontation. These patients are not sociopathic, nor do they usually manifest psychiatric disorders.

298. The answer is C. *(Kaplan, ed 4. pp 151–152.)* Phobias can exist in association with schizophrenic decompensation and may be the initial manifestation of obsessions. People who have anorexia nervosa have phobic fears of losing control of their eating habits and becoming fat. Phobic attacks can be a major aspect in depersonalization states, as exemplified by the phobic anxiety-depersonalization syndrome. Phobias are not likely to be associated with sociopathic personality disorders.

299. The answer is D. *(Kaplan, ed 4. pp 476–477.)* Adjustment disorders are characterized by temporary maladaptive behavior or symptom patterns that are markedly out of proportion to the precipitating stress or stresses. Onset of the disorder may not be coincident with occurrence of the precipitating stressful event, and symptoms may continue well beyond the cessation of the stress. Disturbances of both emotion and conduct may occur in association with adjustment disorders. This diagnosis, however, should not be made when other, specific psychiatric disorders are clearly present.

300. The answer is B. *(Kaplan, ed 4. pp 372–375.)* Suicide attempts are rare in children who develop antisocial personality disorder in adulthood. These children seem to act out their problems in ways other than self-destruction. Theft, incorrigibility, truancy, running away, bad companions, staying out late, and physical aggression all are associated commonly with children who become antisocial adults.

301. The answer is D. *(Kaplan, ed 4. pp 544–545.)* The major characteristic of Ganser's syndrome is that affected persons respond to questions in an appropriate form—as if they understood the questions—but at the same time give absolutely incorrect answers. Thus, rather than being unrelated to the questions asked, these responses may be thought to parallel the correct responses; in fact, Ganser's syndrome may be mistaken for dementia, until the parallelism of these responses is discerned. The syndrome, which is considered to be a disorder of thought and speech, may be a subtype of malingering. It was first described in prison inmates, most of whom were awaiting trial for murder.

302. The answer is A. *(American Psychiatric Association, ed 3-R. pp 269–272. Michels, vol 1, chap 39, pp 8–10.)* Descriptions of multiple personalities in the psychiatric literature are often colorful and dramatic, yet many psychiatrists remain skeptical about the occurrence of this disorder. Multiple personality disorder is currently classified in *DSM III-R* as a type of dissociative disorder. One factor that may lead clinicians to be skeptical about the occurrence of the disorder is that it is frequently not recognized. In the disorder the afflicted person takes on other personalities that the "host" personality is unaware of. As a result the afflicted person may be told of events or behavior that he or she cannot remember. Objects may be found in the person's possession that cannot be accounted for. The diagnosis may be facilitated by hypnosis and might be considered if marked changes in behavior are noted by others.

303. The answer is E (all). *(Michels, vol 1, chap 15, p 11.)* The advantages of multidimensional self-reported instruments, like the MMPI, are that they provide useful supplemental information for the clinician and assist in diagnostic and treatment decision-making. They are cost-effective and can now be done on computer monitors, thereby greatly diminishing inter-rater bias.

304. The answer is D (4). *(American Psychiatric Association, ed 3-R. pp 339–342.)* In schizotypal personality disorder there are not only deficits in interpersonal relatedness, but peculiarities of ideation, appearance, and behavior beginning by early adulthood. These peculiarities are not a part of the diagnosis of schizoid personality disorder. In both conditions there may be constricted affect, but in schizotypal personality disorder the affect may also be quite inappropriate. People with either disorder tend not to have close relationships and to be uncomfortable in social situations.

305. The answer is B (1, 3). *(Michels, vol 1, chap 15, pp 5–6.)* The MMPI and CAQ are empirically based tests of personality. They are scored by matching the subject's responses to those of people with known disorders or traits. The TAT is a projective test in which the subject interprets a series of pictures. The POMS assesses a subject's current mood state via rating how the subject feels in regard to mood adjectives.

306. The answer is D (4). *(Michels, vol 1, chap 15, pp 8–11.)* The circumplex model is a two-dimensional circular ordering of ideas or concepts based on their similarities. For over 30 years it has been used to describe the structure of personality traits. Theoretically, traits close in proximity within the circle are similar, whereas those opposite one another represent bipolarities.

307. The answer is E (all). *(Talbott, p 761.)* Patients with bulimia nervosa engage in self-induced vomiting or use of laxatives or diuretics. They are susceptible to the development of hypokalemic alkalosis and other electrolyte disturbances. These disturbances may induce cardiac arrhythmia, and this can lead to cardiac arrest. Parotid gland enlargement, with elevated serum amylase levels, is common in patients who binge and vomit. Gastric dilatation is a rare complication in patients who binge and should be considered an emergency condition.

308. The answer is C (2, 4). *(Kaplan, ed 4. pp 361–362.)* DSM III-R describes personality disorders as deeply ingrained, inflexible, maladaptive patterns of relating to, perceiving, and thinking about the environment and oneself that result in impairment in adaptive functioning or subjective distress. They are pervasive personality traits and are generally recognized by the time of adolescence or earlier and continue throughout most of adult life.

309. The answer is D (4). *(Kaplan, ed 4. pp 378–380.)* People with dependent personality disorder typically get others to assume major responsibility for their lives. They genuinely appear to lack self-confidence and tend to subordinate their needs to the needs of those on whom they depend. Because they generally are passive, pessimistic, and highly suggestible—traits common to many psychiatrically ill persons—the diagnosis of dependent personality disorder should be made only when these traits are characteristic of long-term functioning.

310. The answer is B (1, 3). *(American Psychiatric Association, ed 3-R. pp 335–336.)* Personality disorders represent a constellation of traits or behaviors that are characteristic of the person's recent and long-term functioning since early adulthood. They are often associated with very significant social and vocational impairment. They are coded on axis II and may coexist with axis I diagnoses.

311. The answer is C (2, 4). *(Kaplan, ed 4. pp 434–437.)* A transsexual is a person who feels a strong incongruity between actual, identified sex and subjective gender identity. Affected persons usually feel trapped in a body of the "wrong" sex and wish to change to the opposite sex. Male transsexualism seems to be divided into two types: "primary" (early-onset), in which men adopt feminine characteristics early in childhood and feel female throughout life; and "secondary" (late-emerging), in which men may be quite masculine and successful in typically masculine roles, such as husband and father. Homosexuality is not necessarily a dominant behavior pattern among transsexuals. Follow-up studies on the efficacy of sex-change surgery for transsexualism are insufficient.

312–314. The answers are: 312-A (1,2,3), 313-E (all), 314-A (1, 2, 3). *(Kaplan, ed 4. pp 499–504. Michels, vol 2, chap 109, pp 1–9.)* Amenorrhea, an altered body image, and an energetic striving for thinness compose the "classic triad" of symptoms and signs of persons who have anorexia nervosa. The often profound cachexia of these persons is usually accompanied by flagrantly distorted ideation about their bodies and by earnest efforts, such as exercising and dieting, to lose what they consider excess weight. In approximately half of all affected girls and women, loss of menstruation occurs before loss of weight. Fear of losing control, lack of concern about loss of menses, constipation, and the classic "good girl" description are other aspects of anorexia nervosa. Among the clinical and laboratory features of anorexia nervosa are bradycardia, leukopenia, hypotension, hypothermia, and elevated serum levels of carotene. Leukopenia, along with malnutrition, may lead to potentially fatal infections. Despite considerable inanition, persons who have this disorder tend to be bright, alert, energetic, and resourceful; in addition, most remain unaware of the life-threatening potential of their disrupted eating habits. Obsessional traits commonly are associated with anorexia nervosa, as is the strong wish to remain passively dependent. Although poor appetite and weight loss may accompany deep depression, underlying depression is unusual in persons affected by anorexia nervosa.

315. The answer is A (1, 2, 3). *(Kaplan, ed 4. p 437.)* Transvestism is defined as persistent, fetishistic cross-dressing occurring exclusively in men. Onset usually is in adolescence. Affected men definitely identify themselves as men (i.e., they are not transsexuals); most are heterosexual, and many are married. Transvestite behavior usually is secret, although at times a willing partner or spouse may participate. For many affected men, cross-dressing provides the only means of sexual arousal. Behavior modification therapy is most likely to succeed with highly motivated men whose fetishes are narrowly defined. Treatment is harder the more a man wishes to pass in public as a woman.

316. The answer is D (4). *(Kaplan, ed 4. pp 545–546.)* Sharing of psychotic symptoms between two persons who are closely tied emotionally defines a folie à deux relationship. Perhaps because of the psychotic nature of their illness, affected persons tend to live in poor socioeconomic environments. The loss of normal emotional ties, increasing insecurity and passivity, dependence, and the possible development of organic disease all make the prognosis of folie à deux worse in geriatric age groups than in others. Treatment of the passive partner of the relationship centers around replacing the dominant participant with a substitute, a long and difficult process that does not always lead to complete recovery. Therapy for the dominant partner involves treatment of the existing psychosis, which usually is schizophrenia.

317. The answer is A (1, 2, 3). *(American Psychiatric Association, ed 3-R. pp 65–67. Kaplan, ed 4. pp 499–500.)* Anorexia nervosa occurs predominantly in women, particularly in adolescents and young adults. It is characterized by an intense fear of obesity, distorted body image, and progressive weight loss. The mortality has not been definitely established but is probably about 10 percent. Current criteria specify that the patient must have lost at least 25 percent of original body weight in order to warrant the diagnosis of anorexia nervosa.

318. The answer is B (1, 3). *(Kaplan, ed 4. pp 552–554.)* People who have Munchausen's syndrome have a remarkable ability to feign serious physical illness. Skilled physicians and other medical professionals are often taken in by the dramatic performances, so that a history of multiple operations is common. Women affected by Munchausen's syndrome often are diagnosed as histrionic, and men who have the disorder frequently are considered psychopathic. Once hospitalized, these patients become hostile and threatening. Treatment of choice is long-term psychotherapy.

319. The answer is A (1, 2, 3). *(Kaplan, ed 4. p 548.)* People who have Capgras' syndrome usually are schizophrenic and delusional. They insist that certain persons in their environment (usually those who are familiar and in some way important to them) are imposters or exact doubles. Cognitive and perceptual processes are disrupted in affected persons; because a feeling of familiarity is missing, true recognition becomes impossible. Capgras' syndrome is similar to false memories of familiarity, such as déjà vu, and to certain aspects of epileptic aura.

320. The answer is B (1, 3). *(Kaplan, ed 4. pp 330–332.)* Persons with paranoid personality disorder are markedly suspicious of others. They are intensely alert to any potential disloyalty, threat, or injustice, and they are typically overconcerned with perceived hidden motives or special meanings in the behavior of others. Although they may be moralistic, self-righteous, and litigious, paranoid persons are acutely sensitive to matters of power and status and are usually contemptuous of the weak and helpless. Because of the nature of their disorder, affected persons usually are very reluctant to enter into psychotherapy. When they do enter therapy, therapists do best by maintaining a carefully professional, somewhat distant attitude. The epidemiology of paranoid personality disorder is not well established. The percentage of affected persons who go on to develop frank schizophrenia is not known.

321. The answer is B (1, 3). *(Kaplan, ed 4. pp 13–14.)* The influence of genetic factors on the development of some specific personality traits is strongly suggested by a number of studies. Introversion and extroversion seem, even in animal studies, to be more under the influence of heredity than environment. In addition, the ability to be sedated by a fixed dose of a hypnotic is apparently higher in outgoing persons than in those who are depressive or introverted. In Danish adoption studies, adoptees born to psychologically healthy parents were found to fare reasonably well even when one or both of their adopted parents had schizophrenia. Whether relatives of people who have obsessive compulsive personality traits are more likely than normal to display these same traits is moot, with studies supporting both sides of the question.

322. The answer is B (1, 3). *(Kaplan, ed 4. pp 372–375.)* People who have antisocial personality disorder often are colorful, superficially charming, and manipulative. In addition, many seem quite intelligent. However, affect typically is not in proportion to behavior—that is, they tend to present bland rationalizations of their actions. Antisocial behavior most often is displayed by teenagers and young adults, with decreasing prevalence rates thereafter. However, up to one-third of persons with antisocial personality disorder become alcoholic. Treatment, which usually involves lengthy, repetitive limit-setting, often is complicated by well-meaning "rescuers" who continually extricate these people from difficulty, allowing them to return promptly to their antisocial ways.

323. The answer is A (1, 2, 3). *(Kaplan, ed 4. pp 381–383.)* Obstructionism, stubbornness, negativism, and deliberate inefficiency are the major personality characteristics of passive aggressive persons. When these people are hospitalized, it is frequently in conjunction with bouts of anxiety, excessive drinking, depression, and resultant stormy interpersonal relationships. People with passive aggressive personality disorder are no more likely than others to develop schizophrenia.

324. The answer is E (all). *(Kaplan, ed 4. pp 479–487.)* Disorders of impulse control involve failure to resist impulses causing harm to self or others. Although the impulse may be premeditated and consciously resisted, it is egosyntonic at the time it is performed—that is, the act fulfills a conscious wish at the moment. Subtypes of the disorder include kleptomania (compulsive stealing), pyromania (compulsive fire-setting), compulsive gambling, intermittent explosive disorder, and isolated explosive episode. Most persons displaying pyromania or intermittent explosive disorder are male. Intermittent explosive disorder usually begins in adolescence or early adulthood and tends to recede by middle age.

325. The answer is D (4). *(Kaplan, ed 4. pp 375–377.)* People who have borderline personality disorder describe intense moods with chronic feelings of emptiness. When in crisis, they are typically intensely angry, and their behavior may be impulsive, unpredictable, and self-destructive. They are dependent in their relationships, which tend to be intense but unstable. They have great difficulty being alone. Identity disturbance, substance abuse, and even brief psychotic episodes may be part of the clinical presentation. Although people with borderline personality disorder may demonstrate ordinary reasoning abilities on structured tests, their responses to unstructured tests are markedly deviant. Regressive psychotherapy should not be employed because these people have great difficulty tolerating any type of intense emotion.

326–330. The answers are: 326-B, 327-C, 328-A, 329-D, 330-B. *(American Psychiatric Association, ed 3-R. pp 339–340, 351–352.)* Patients with avoidant and schizoid personality disorders share the trait of having few close personal attachments. However, while the schizoid person is emotionally cold and aloof with an absence of tender feelings for others and indifference to praise or criticism, the avoidant person is hypersensitive to rejection and desirous of affection and acceptance, but unwilling to enter into relationships for fear of rejection. Neither are characterized by eccentricities of speech or behavior, as seen in the schizotypal personality. Even though both avoidant and schizoid persons will not have many personal relationships, the avoidant person experiences much more psychic pain than does the schizoid person. This is a key differential feature.

Alcoholism and Substance Abuse

DIRECTIONS: Each question below contains five suggested responses. Select the **one best** response to each question.

331. In people with normal liver function, alcohol is metabolized at

(A) 0.5 ounce per hour
(B) 1 ounce per hour
(C) 5 ounces per hour
(D) 0.5 ounce per minute
(E) 1 ounce per minute

332. Another primary psychiatric illness should be seriously considered if a psychosis, precipitated by ingestion of a hallucinogen, should persist beyond

(A) 2 hours
(B) 24 hours
(C) 48 hours
(D) 2 weeks
(E) 6 weeks

333. Task impairment begins when the blood alcohol level reaches

(A) 0.1 percent
(B) 0.5 percent
(C) 1 percent
(D) 5 percent
(E) 10 percent

334. Death can occur at a serum alcohol level of

(A) 30 mg per 100 ml
(B) 200 mg per 100 ml
(C) 500 mg per 100 ml
(D) 800 mg per 100 ml
(E) 1000 mg per 100 ml

Questions 335–337

A 35-year-old man stumbles into the emergency room. His pulse is 100, his blood pressure is 170/95, and he is diaphoretic. He is tremulous and has difficulty relating a history. He does admit to insomnia the past two nights and thinks a curtain is a ghost in the room. He also states he is a drinker since age 19, but has not had a drink in 4 days.

335. The most likely diagnosis is

(A) adjustment disorder
(B) atypical psychosis
(C) alcohol withdrawal delirium (delirium tremens)
(D) alcohol intoxication
(E) alcohol idiosyncratic intoxication

336. Initial drug treatment should include

(A) haloperidol 10 mg IM
(B) chlorpromazine 50 mg IM
(C) lithium 300 mg PO
(D) chlordiazepoxide 50 mg PO
(E) imipramine 50 mg PO

337. Appropriate follow-up treatment for this patient would include all the following EXCEPT

(A) complete history and physical examination with emphasis on hepatic, gastrointestinal, and neurologic functioning
(B) psychological assessment to determine underlying psychopathology
(C) social assessment to identify social/environmental stressors contributing to the problem
(D) referral to alcoholics anonymous (AA)
(E) fluphenazine decanoate (Prolixin) 1 ml IM with an appointment to his local mental health clinic for follow-up

338. All the following drugs used to treat heroin addiction are narcotic antagonists EXCEPT

(A) naltrexone
(B) cyclazocine
(C) methadone (Dolophine)
(D) levallorphan tartrate (Lorfan)
(E) naloxone (Narcan)

339. A 59-year-old man comes to a hospital for an elective herniorrhaphy. Except for revealing mild hyperreflexia and several healed scalp lacerations, the initial physical examination is normal. The nursing staff reports that the man has been somewhat irritable and that he slept poorly before surgery and complained of bad dreams the next day. On the day after his successful surgery—about 72 hours after admission—the man goes berserk. Frightened and disoriented, he says that his skin is crawling with spiders; he does not recognize the nursing staff or his doctor. He insists he is in a prison camp and that the walls are closing in on him. Despite attempts by the staff to soothe him, he attempts to "escape." A cursory physical examination at this time reveals flushing, tremulousness, and injected conjunctivae. Rectal temperature is 38.3°C (101°F), and pulse is rapid, irregular, and thready. He is perspiring freely. Neurological examination shows marked hyperreflexia (but no clonus), tremor, and agitation. He is disoriented to time and place.

All the following statements about this man's disorder are true EXCEPT that

(A) with proper treatment, this disorder usually resolves in 3 to 10 days
(B) hospitalization probably triggered onset of this disorder
(C) the disorder, even if untreated, will not cause death
(D) convulsions may occur if this disorder is untreated
(E) assessment of hydration and nutritional status and electrolyte balance is important

340. All the following statements about alcoholism are true EXCEPT

(A) current classifications of alcoholic disorders are based on etiological factors
(B) the consequences, rather than the actual amount, of drinking may be the best means for detecting alcoholism
(C) cultural background may affect the incidence of alcoholism
(D) the tendency for alcoholism to run in families is a well-established observation
(E) the reported incidence of alcoholism in women is substantially lower than in men

341. A 39-year-old man enters an emergency room complaining of anxiety and extreme sleeplessness. He is noted to be markedly tremulous, and while being examined he has a grand mal seizure. This man might be suffering from withdrawal from any of the following substances EXCEPT

(A) alcohol
(B) haloperidol (Haldol)
(C) meprobamate (Equanil and Miltown)
(D) phenobarbital
(E) diazepam (Valium)

342. Delirium tremens, which can develop in persons who abstain from drinking after a prolonged period of alcohol use, is characteristically associated with all the following EXCEPT

(A) bradycardia
(B) tremor
(C) vivid visual hallucinations
(D) disorientation to time and place
(E) a course of 3 to 7 days

DIRECTIONS: Each question below contains four suggested responses of which **one or more** is correct. Select

A	if	**1, 2, and 3**	are correct
B	if	**1 and 3**	are correct
C	if	**2 and 4**	are correct
D	if	**4**	is correct
E	if	**1, 2, 3, and 4**	are correct

343. Symptoms suggesting schizophrenia are seen in the use of which of the following substances?

(1) Cocaine
(2) LSD
(3) Amphetamines
(4) Mescaline

344. Intoxication with cocaine in the chronic user may be associated with

(1) paranoid psychosis
(2) hyperreflexia and seizures
(3) euphoria and pressured speech
(4) tachycardia and mydriasis

345. Diagnostic criteria for alcohol dependence include which of the following?

(1) A pattern of pathological alcohol use
(2) Impairment in social or occupational functioning due to alcohol use
(3) A need for increased amounts of alcohol to achieve the desired effect
(4) Development of withdrawal symptoms after stopping or reducing drinking

346. The major physiologic effects of cocaine include high-potency

(1) local anesthetic action
(2) sympathomimetic action
(3) stimulation of the central nervous system
(4) vasodilatation, producing hypotension

347. The withdrawal syndrome that can occur in persons who suddenly stop taking amphetamines in large doses is characterized by

(1) seizures
(2) hunger
(3) insomnia
(4) depression

348. Signs of pathological alcohol use or impairment in functioning can be useful for diagnosis of alcohol abuse or alcohol dependence. Examples include which of the following?

(1) Need for daily alcohol in order to function
(2) Absenteeism from work
(3) Blackouts
(4) Intoxication more than twice a year

SUMMARY OF DIRECTIONS

A	B	C	D	E
1,2,3	1,3	2,4	4	All are
only	only	only	only	correct

349. Drugs that can produce a psychosis whose symptoms are strikingly similar to paranoid schizophrenia include

(1) cocaine
(2) methylphenidate
(3) amphetamines
(4) propranolol

350. Abuse of glue and other volatile solvents can be described by which of the following statements?

(1) Glue sniffing is most common in children and teenagers
(2) Glue sniffing leads to intoxication similar to that caused by alcohol, and amnesia for the episode may occur
(3) Inhaling volatile substances can cause irreversible damage to brain, liver, and kidneys
(4) Inhaling volatile substances can result in death due to respiratory arrest

351. Intoxication with phencyclidine (PCP) is characteristically associated with

(1) vertical and horizontal nystagmus
(2) hypotension
(3) myoclonus and ataxia
(4) sedation

352. The Wernicke-Korsakoff syndrome can be described by which of the following statements?

(1) It usually is associated with chronic alcoholism
(2) Remote, not recent, memory is impaired
(3) Ophthalmoplegia, nystagmus, and ataxia are common
(4) Treatment of choice is niacin

353. Correct statements about alcohol abuse in the United States include which of the following?

(1) It is the second most serious drug-abuse problem
(2) During the 15 years prior to 1980 the per capita consumption of alcohol increased markedly
(3) A cause-and-effect relationship exists between the amount of alcohol consumed and the incidence of alcoholism
(4) Approximately 10 million people are alcoholic

354. The neuropsychiatric changes often associated with meperidine (Demerol) include

(1) serene detachment
(2) dysphoria and irritability
(3) cataplexy
(4) myoclonic twitches

355. Correct statements about cocaine include which of the following?

(1) It is usually taken orally
(2) Onset of intoxication is typically slow, over a 3- to 4-hour period, and includes euphoria and elation as major features
(3) Withdrawal from cocaine must be done slowly in a hospital setting
(4) After the high, a person often feels depressed, anxious, and irritable, leading to desire for further use of the drug

356. The treatment of opiate addiction can be described by which of the following statements?

(1) Medication is often used in the detoxification phase of treatment
(2) Methadyl acetate (*l*-acetylmethadol) is similar to methadone but its therapeutic effects last longer
(3) Methadone is popular in the maintenance treatment of narcotic addiction because of its ability to block the euphoric effects of narcotic drugs
(4) Narcotic antagonists are used for treating heroin overdose but not for preventing and treating narcotic addiction

357. Disulfiram can be described by which of the following statements?

(1) Its use is absolutely contraindicated in persons with heart disease
(2) It may lead to toxic accumulation of phenytoin (Dilantin) in persons taking both medications
(3) It is metabolized rapidly
(4) When taken with alcohol, it can produce nausea, flushing, and hypotension

358. True statements regarding alcohol withdrawal phenomena include which of the following?

(1) The appearance of an alcohol withdrawal seizure most likely indicates the onset of delirium tremens
(2) Alcohol withdrawal seizures generally occur about 12 hours after the last drink and can be prevented by the use of anticonvulsant medication
(3) Alcoholic hallucinosis is characterized by persistent olfactory hallucinations after the withdrawal is completed
(4) Alcoholic hallucinosis is associated with an intact sensorium

359. True statements about alcohol idiosyncratic intoxication (pathological intoxication) include which of the following?

(1) It usually begins slowly
(2) It occurs after a large alcohol intake
(3) It involves vivid recall ("flashbacks") for the period of time involved
(4) It may involve aggressive behavior toward self and others

DIRECTIONS: The group of questions below consists of lettered headings followed by a set of numbered items. For each numbered item select the **one** lettered heading with which it is **most** closely associated. Each lettered heading may be used **once, more than once, or not at all.**

Questions 360–363

Match the following.

(A) Tolerance
(B) Potentiation
(C) Withdrawal
(D) Dependence
(E) Addiction

360. A repertoire of behaviors that maintain drug use

361. A larger dose of the drug is required to obtain the same effect

362. A physiological state that follows cessation of or reduction in drug use

363. A syndrome of clinically significant symptoms following cessation of substance use

Alcoholism and Substance Abuse

Answers

331. The answer is B. *(Kaplan, ed 4. p 417.)* For the average healthy person, alcohol is metabolized at the rate of 1 ounce of alcoholic drink per hour. Other factors that will influence the blood alcohol level include prior drinking history, body size, and the amount of food in the stomach. There is a range in the rate at which alcohol is metabolized by the liver. The rate is determined by the activity of the enzyme alcohol dehydrogenase and varies among cultural and ethnic groups.

332. The answer is D. *(Stoudemire, p 249.)* Most cases of intoxication with a hallucinogen are over within several hours. But prolonged drug-induced psychoses may occur, especially with PCP, in which the psychosis may last 2 to 7 days. In some instances the drug appears to precipitate a latent psychotic illness, and if the psychosis persists beyond 2 weeks this should be seriously considered.

333. The answer is B. *(Kaplan, ed 4. p 416.)* Most people become significantly uncoordinated when their blood alcohol level reaches 0.1 percent. Research has shown task impairment to begin at blood alcohol levels of about 0.5 percent. Blood alcohol level is influenced by the amount of alcohol as well as by body weight.

334. The answer is D. *(Kaplan, ed 4. p 417.)* An inexperienced drinker can show signs of intoxication at 30 mg per 100 ml; virtually everyone is intoxicated at a level of 200 mg per 100 ml. Unconsciousness usually occurs at a level of 500 mg per 100 ml and death usually occurs between 600 and 800 mg per 100 ml. Unconsciousness usually occurs before one can drink enough to die.

335–337. The answers are: 335-C, 336-D, 337-E. *(Kaplan, ed 4. pp 416–419.)* Alcohol withdrawal delirium (delerium tremens) is the severest form of alcohol withdrawal. Five percent of all hospitalized alcoholics develop delirium tremens during their hospital course. Clinically, delerium tremens develops 2 to 7 days after cessation of drinking and is characterized by tachycardia, diaphoresis, hypertension, confusion, insomnia, illusions or visual hallucinations, and tremor. Delirium tremens is most common in people with at least a 5-year drinking history in which binges are common. Initial treatment should include chlordiazepoxide 50 to 100 mg. Phenothiazines should not be used because of neurologic problems and probable preexisting hepatic impairment. Follow-up treatment should include a complete bio-psychosocial evaluation. AA is an excellent referral source.

338. The answer is C. *(Kaplan, ed 4. pp 394–398.)* Dependence on heroin and other opiates can be treated with narcotic antagonists, such as cyclazocine, naloxone (Narcan), naltrexone, and levallorphan tartrate (Lorfan). These agents, which are not addictive, block the action of opiate compounds, thus curtailing their effects. Methadone (Dolophine) is a drug whose pharmacological properties are similar to those of morphine. The chronic administration of methadone produces both tolerance and physical dependence. By inducing tolerance to opiatelike drugs, methadone is thought to block the euphoric effects of "street" narcotics, such as heroin.

339. The answer is C. *(Kaplan, ed 4. pp 419–420.)* The most likely diagnosis for the man described in the question is delirium tremens, an acute psychotic state associated with chronic alcoholism and most often observed in persons older than 30 years of age. If treated properly, affected persons recover in 3 to 10 days; if they are untreated, the mortality may reach 15 percent. Death also can result from oversedation. Delirium tremens in the postoperative patient can be mistaken for a postsurgical complication, in that irritability, diaphoresis, tachycardia, and fever can be common to both conditions. Epileptiform seizures also can occur in association with delirium tremens. Hospitalization may have precipitated this condition in the man described in the question because it imposed a period of abstinence from alcohol.

340. The answer is A. *(Kaplan, ed 4. pp 414–416.)* Existing classifications of alcoholic disorders are predominantly descriptive; in most cases the etiology is obscure. The best means of detecting alcoholism is by being alert to the possibility in persons presenting with frequently occurring sequelae—physical, social, and psychological—of alcohol abuse. Cultural, ethnic, and social factors seem to affect prevalence rates of alcoholism; in some immigrant groups, the characteristic rate of alcoholism may persist for several generations in the United States, before equaling the national norm. It is well established that alcoholism tends to run in families. More men than women still are reported to be alcoholic, but this discrepancy may reflect in part the fact that women are able to "hide" their alcohol problem with less difficulty.

341. The answer is B. *(Kaplan, ed 4. p 27.)* Haloperidol (Haldol) is an antipsychotic agent of the butyrophenone class. It does not produce the classic physical dependence and withdrawal effects that are associated with alcohol and antianxiety agents, such as diazepam, meprobamate (Equanil and Miltown), and phenobarbital. As in the case described in the question, symptoms of withdrawal from these agents can include tremor, insomnia, and seizures.

342. The answer is A. *(Kaplan, ed 4. pp 419–420.)* Delirium tremens can occur when a person stops drinking after prolonged use of alcohol. It is a hypermetabolic state that is associated with tachycardia, fever, tremulousness, and increased blood pressure. Affected persons are confused, are disoriented to time and place, and often have visual, tactile, or olfactory hallucinations. Symptoms usually last from 3 to 7 days. The mortality is significant in untreated persons.

343. The answer is E (all). *(Talbott, pp 339–343.)* Cocaine, LSD, amphetamines, and mescaline can all present with clinical symptoms suggesting schizophrenia. Perceptual disturbances including hallucinations, delusions (particularly paranoid), and illusions are commonly seen in drug abusers. An important factor in helping to make the differential diagnosis is that substance abusers usually experience visual hallucinations, while schizophrenics complain of auditory hallucinations.

344. The answer is E (all). *(Stoudemire, p 248.)* Intoxication with cocaine is usually characterized by subjective feelings of euphoria, elation, excitement, and restlessness. The patient often displays pressured speech, and on examination there are signs of the sympathetic stimulation. These signs include tachycardia, mydriasis, and sweating. With chronic use one may see suspiciousness or frank paranoid psychosis. When intoxication is at the overdose level, hyperpyrexia, hyperreflexia, and seizures result. Ultimately there may be progression to coma and respiratory arrest. Cardiac arrhythmias may be associated with sudden death.

345. The answer is E (all). *(Kaplan, ed 4. p 415.)* Alcohol dependence is described by *DSM III-R* as the pathological use of alcohol resulting in impaired social or occupational functioning. The need for daily drinking in order to function adequately and an inability to cut down or stop characterizes pathologic use, along with blackouts and continued drinking despite serious physical disorders related to drinking. For the diagnosis to be made, either tolerance or withdrawal symptoms must be evident. Tolerance is the need for increased amounts of alcohol to achieve the desired effect or a marked diminished effect with the same amount, and withdrawal is physical symptoms (such as morning shaking) with reduction or cessation of drinking.

346. The answer is A (1, 2, 3). *(Stoudemire, p 248.)* Cocaine is a high-potency local anesthetic that appears to work by blocking nerve impulses through its effect on sodium conduction of nerve cell membranes. It is also a potent sympathomimetic, potentiating the actions of catecholamines in the autonomic nervous system. This results in the characteristic tachycardia, vasoconstriction, and hypertension. The agitation and arousal effects are largely due to the stimulation of the central nervous system via potentiation of the actions of such neurotransmitters as dopamine and norepinephrine.

347. The answer is C (2, 4). *(Gilman, ed 7. pp 553–554. Kaplan, ed 4. pp 164–165.)* Withdrawal from heavy amphetamine abuse is characterized by drug craving, fatigue, increased sleep, headache, cramps, and hunger. Depression may be quite profound and can lead to suicide attempts. Seizures are not a feature of amphetamine withdrawal.

348. The answer is A (1, 2, 3). *(American Psychiatric Association, ed 3-R. pp 173–175.)* A pattern of pathological alcohol use includes a need for daily use of alcohol for adequate functioning, inability to cut down or stop drinking, repeated efforts to control or reduce excess drinking by "going on the wagon" (periods of temporary abstinence) or restricting drinking to certain times of the day, binges (remaining intoxicated throughout the day for at least 2 days), occasional consumption of a fifth of spirits (or its equivalent in wine or beer), amnesic periods for events occurring while intoxicated (blackouts), continuation of drinking despite a serious physical disorder that the person knows is exacerbated by alcohol use, and drinking of nonbeverage alcohol. Impairment in social or occupational functioning as the result of alcohol use might include violence while intoxicated, absence from work, loss of job, legal difficulties (e.g., arrest for intoxicated behavior, traffic accidents while intoxicated), arguments, or difficulties with family or friends because of excessive alcohol use.

349. The answer is A (1, 2, 3). *(Stoudemire, pp 248–249.)* An "amphetamine psychosis," with symptoms strikingly similar to those seen in paranoid schizophrenia, can be seen in chronic abuse of cocaine or other sympathomimetic agents, such as amphetamines, methylphenidate, and other stimulants. The manifestations include agitation, paranoia, delusions, and hallucinations. Propranolol and haloperidol are among the drugs reported as useful in overdose.

350. The answer is E (all). *(Kaplan, ed 4. p 410.)* Glue is a favorite substance of abuse among children and teenagers. Intoxication can produce aggressive behavior, hallucinations, and amnesia for the acute period. Other volatile substances, such as toluene, lacquers, and paint thinners, are particularly dangerous because of the risk of tissue damage from repeated use. Death from overdose can occur.

351. The answer is B (1, 3). *(Stoudemire, p 249.)* Patients intoxicated with PCP often present because of violence and bizarre, excited behavior. On examination one frequently encounters eye signs such as horizontal and vertical nystagmus. Myoclonus and ataxia are also common. Physical examination usually demonstrates the presence of tachycardia and hypertension.

352. The answer is B (1, 3). *(Kaplan, ed 4. p 420.)* The Wernicke-Korsakoff syndrome, which most often is associated with chronic alcoholism, has two components: Wernicke's encephalopathy and Korsakoff's psychosis. Symptoms of

Wernicke's disease include ophthalmoplegia, nystagmus, ataxia, and confusion. Korsakoff's psychosis, which usually follows the encephalopathy, involves severe impairment of recent memory. Thiamine is the treatment of choice for the Wernicke-Korsakoff syndrome.

353. The answer is C (2, 4). *(Kaplan, ed 4. p 414.)* Alcoholism is clearly the most serious drug-abuse problem in the United States. In 1974, a federal report estimated the number of cases of alcoholism to be 9 million. The rate of consumption of alcohol in this country was nearly one-third higher in 1980 than it was in 1964. Although it is thought that higher alcohol consumption means a higher prevalence rate of alcoholism in a given country, a cause-and-effect relationship has yet to be shown.

354. The answer is C (2, 4). *(Hales, pp 162, 171–172).* The adverse changes associated with meperidine use are commonly dysphoria, irritability, and myoclonic twitches. As toxicity increases with the accumulation of the metabolite normeperidine, there may be seizures and delirium. This picture is often seen in medical and surgical patients being treated for pain. The condition is treated by changing to another narcotic, such as morphine, at an equianalgesic dosage.

355. The answer is D (4). *(Kaplan, ed 4. pp 405–406.)* The most common intake of cocaine is by application to the nasal membrane (''snorting''). Other routes include smoking and the intravenous route (''skin popping''). Sniffing may lead to perforations in the nasal septum. Cocaine is inactivated when taken orally. The onset of intoxication is quite rapid; symptoms like euphoria and elation begin within 1 hour and are usually entirely over within 24 hours. The ''crash'' after intoxication often exacerbates further drug use. Withdrawal from cocaine is not dangerous medically, so use can be stopped abruptly.

356. The answer is A (1, 2, 3). *(Kaplan, ed 4. pp 486–487.)* Medication frequently is used to help narcotic-addicted people through the withdrawal process. The most widely used medication is methadone; in programs of methadone maintenance, the drug must be taken on a daily basis. A methadone derivative, methadyl acetate (*l*-acetylmethadol), effectively blocks the euphoric effects of opiates for 2 to 3 days, and the search is continuing for even longer-lasting substitutes. Although their main usefulness is in the treatment of narcotic overdose through their ability to displace opiates from receptors, narcotic antagonists also have been used in the prevention and treatment of narcotic addiction. Unlike methadone, narcotic antagonists do not themselves exert narcotic effects and thus are not addictive.

357. The answer is C (2, 4). *(Kaplan, ed 4. p 426.)* Disulfiram, when taken with alcohol, can lead to nausea, flushing, dizziness, palpitations, hypotension, air hunger, and a sense of apprehension. Because the drug is metabolized slowly, these effects can occur if alcohol is ingested as long as 4 days after stopping the medication. Caution should be exercised when giving disulfiram to persons who have heart disease because hypotension can develop as a result of the disulfiram-alcohol reaction; however, heart disease is not an absolute contraindication. Use of the drug has been associated with accumulation of toxic levels of phenytoin (Dilantin) and related medications.

358. The answer is D (4). *(Kaplan, ed 4. p 418.)* Grand mal seizures occur infrequently as a complication of alcohol withdrawal, with or without delirium tremens. These generalized seizures usually appear within 48 hours after drinking has stopped and cease without any specific treatment. The current thinking is that anticonvulsant medication is ineffective in treating or preventing alcohol withdrawal seizures. Alcoholic hallucinosis is characterized by auditory hallucinations that persist even after a person withdrawing from alcohol has otherwise become symptom-free. Alcoholic hallucinosis, in contrast to delirium tremens, is associated with an intact sensorium.

359. The answer is D (4). *(Kaplan, ed 4. pp 417–418.)* Alcohol idiosyncratic intoxication (pathological intoxication) is a condition in which a person, usually of a younger age, after drinking a very small amount of alcohol, behaves as though he or she had drunk a great deal more. The onset is typically sudden and dramatic, often with aggressive behavior toward self or others. The episode may last minutes to hours and is often followed by a period of sleep and then amnesia for the episode. This is an uncommon condition, and patients must be assisted in achieving abstinence to avoid further episodes.

360–363. The answers are: 360-E, 361-A, 362-C, 363-D. *(Stoudemire, pp 237–238.)* These terms are commonly confused or used ambiguously. Tolerance refers to a pharmacologic effect in which a larger dose of a drug becomes necessary over time to achieve the same effect. Dependence is a condition in which withdrawal symptoms occur if the drug is stopped, and these symptoms indicate loss of control and usually lead to further drug use despite adverse consequences. The term addiction is often confused with dependence and refers to a whole repertoire of behaviors that serve to maintain drug use. With respect to drugs of abuse, one may see both tolerance and dependence simultaneously. The addicted person is one who has a whole series of behaviors and other phenomena that span the spectrum of the bio-psychosocial structure of human existence. For this reason, successful treatment programs must be very broad in their approach to the patient's biological, psychological and social problems.

Psychotherapies

DIRECTIONS: Each question below contains five suggested responses. Select the **one best** response to each question.

364. In psychoanalytic theory, the phenomenon of transference

(A) occurs only in the relationship between the therapist and the patient
(B) impedes the progress of therapy because it distorts reality
(C) makes it difficult to reconstruct the patient's past
(D) involves the unconscious imposition of the experience of a past relationship onto a present one
(E) is manifested primarily in the patient's dreams

365. The major therapeutic techniques employed in cognitive psychotherapy include all the following EXCEPT

(A) "collaborative empiricism"
(B) interpretation of unconscious motivation
(C) behavioral techniques
(D) identification of irrational beliefs and automatic thoughts
(E) identification of attitudes underlying negatively biased thoughts

366. Of the following, the most sophisticated test of neurologically based cognitive impairment is the

(A) Rorschach
(B) Bender-Gestalt
(C) Minnesota multiphasic personality inventory
(D) Halstead-Reitan
(E) Hamilton rating scale

367. The psychotherapy of personality disorders is made more difficult by the fact that character traits are usually

(A) ego-dystonic
(B) ego-syntonic
(C) unrelated to conflict
(D) so difficult to identify
(E) unrecognized by important persons in the patient's life

368. All the following are true statements about supportive psychotherapy EXCEPT

(A) regressive transference is encouraged and interpreted
(B) it is generally used for healthy persons in crisis or for patients with ego deficits
(C) a major goal is to support reality testing
(D) suggestion and reassurance are employed
(E) there is an attempt to strengthen defenses

369. Psychotherapy of stress-response syndromes most commonly

(A) emphasizes early intervention
(B) involves long-term psychodynamic psychotherapy
(C) uses antidepressant medication to relieve despondency and grief responses to acute loss
(D) encourages patients to maintain their normal activities during the acute phase
(E) avoids attention to preexisting conflicts and developmental difficulties that rendered the person unusually vulnerable

370. Erik Erikson's concept of the life cycle is characterized by all the following EXCEPT

(A) eight states of ego development
(B) the epigenetic principle
(C) phase-specific developmental crisis
(D) personality development completed by the end of adolescence
(E) generativity

371. A woman with anorgasmia is undergoing sex therapy as originally described by Masters and Johnson. All the following statements about her treatment are true EXCEPT

(A) the treatment would include readings and explanations regarding sexuality
(B) the woman might be encouraged to achieve orgasm by masturbating herself
(C) the husband would not be allowed to participate in the therapy sessions until late in the treatment
(D) the patient would be instructed not to have intercourse early on in treatment
(E) the approach is strongly behavioral in its orientation

372. In order to be treated successfully in psychoanalysis, a neurotic patient must have all the following attributes EXCEPT

(A) a reservoir of basic trust
(B) a capacity for reality testing
(C) a capacity for internalization
(D) an ability to tolerate a dependent position
(E) a minimum age of 20 years

373. Traditional psychoanalysis is commonly used in the treatment of persons affected by all the following conditions EXCEPT

(A) conversion disorders
(B) obsessive compulsive disorders
(C) personality disorders
(D) psychotic disorders
(E) certain perversions

374. All the following statements about interpersonal psychotherapy, as developed by Klerman and his colleagues, are true EXCEPT

(A) it is a short-term psychotherapy
(B) it is often combined with medication
(C) it was developed to treat patients with nonpsychotic major depression
(D) the primary emphasis is on conjoint treatment of couples and group psychotherapy
(E) it aims to improve interpersonal communication

375. If a person is late for therapy four times in a row, the therapist should

(A) make up the time at the end of the hour
(B) admonish the patient
(C) try to elicit the meaning of the behavior
(D) ignore the behavior
(E) refer the patient to another therapist

376. An appropriate therapeutic attitude toward the schizophrenic patient includes all the following EXCEPT

(A) respect for the patient's need for privacy
(B) a consistent approach to the patient
(C) a desire to rescue the patient
(D) a focus on the patient's assets as well as on the patient's pathology
(E) tolerance of negative or bizarre behaviors

377. In general, group therapy is intended to enable individuals to do all the following EXCEPT

(A) learn new models of behavior
(B) discover that their problems are not unique
(C) develop a sense of belonging
(D) develop "basic trust"
(E) change their behavior to comply with group models

378. Group therapy is LEAST effective for individuals who have

(A) major mood disorders
(B) paranoid disorders
(C) personality disorders
(D) neuroses
(E) schizophrenia

DIRECTIONS: Each question below contains four suggested responses of which **one or more** is correct. Select

A	if	**1, 2, and 3**	are correct
B	if	**1 and 3**	are correct
C	if	**2 and 4**	are correct
D	if	**4**	is correct
E	if	**1, 2, 3, and 4**	are correct

379. Correct statements regarding biofeedback include that it

(1) usually employs instrumentation
(2) is designed to facilitate self-regulation of bodily processes
(3) may be used to modify brain wave frequencies
(4) is an effective treatment for fecal incontinence

380. True statements regarding hypnosis include that it is

(1) associated with sleep electrophysiology, using EEG criteria
(2) a form of intense, focused alertness
(3) a treatment method first employed by Freud
(4) possible with the majority of psychiatric outpatients

381. The cognitive model of depression holds that the majority of depressed patients

(1) take a chronically negative view of themselves
(2) interpret life experience in a predominantly negative way
(3) look to the future in a pessimistic way
(4) have symptoms and affects derived from negative cognitive schema

382. Treatments commonly used in agoraphobia include

(1) administration of tricyclic antidepressants
(2) psychotherapy
(3) behavior modification
(4) administration of monoamine oxidase (MAO) inhibitors

383. People who have homosexual feelings or fantasies

(1) are regarded as pathological by mental health professionals
(2) have an axis I diagnosis of homosexuality in *DSM III-R*
(3) show much more psychopathology than persons with exclusively heterosexual fantasies
(4) may be married and exclusively heterosexual in their behavior

384. A young married woman, who was incestuously abused as a child, seeks treatment for depression. Which of the following symptoms might this woman experience?

(1) Sexual dysfunction
(2) Marital difficulties
(3) Intense guilt
(4) Physical and emotional abuse toward her children

385. Placebos have been shown to

(1) be frequently effective in the treatment of endogenous depression
(2) be frequently effective in the treatment of neurotic symptoms
(3) be frequently effective in controlling the primary symptoms of schizophrenia
(4) have potentially significant side effects when used to treat persons with psychiatric disorders

386. Correct statements concerning hypnosis include which of the following?

(1) Hypnosis is a sleep-related state
(2) Individual susceptibility to hypnosis can be determined only by attempting to induce a trance
(3) Hypnotizability tends to increase with the degree of psychopathology
(4) Hypnosis is a relatively safe procedure

387. Studies of individual outpatient psychotherapy of schizophrenia have shown that

(1) psychotherapy does more harm than good
(2) psychotherapy alone is significantly less effective than antipsychotic drug treatment alone
(3) psychotherapy almost never has any effect on outcome
(4) psychotherapy plus drug treatment is most effective in preventing relapse

388. Systematic desensitization involves

(1) relaxation training
(2) hierarchy construction
(3) imagined scenes
(4) exploration of conflict

389. The management of the hospitalized suicidal patient includes which of the following?

(1) Continuous observation by staff
(2) Removal of all harmful objects
(3) Inservice education on the management of suicidal patients
(4) Special focus on bathroom activities

390. Existential psychotherapy is associated with

(1) a search for the meaning of a person's life
(2) an emphasis on past development
(3) spiritual values
(4) a theory of psychopathology

391. Day hospital programs play an important therapeutic role as

(1) an alternative to inpatient care
(2) a transition from inpatient care
(3) an alternative to outpatient care
(4) an alternative to nursing home care for the elderly

392. Correct statements about transference neurosis include which of the following?

(1) It begins clinically as a decreased preoccupation with analysis
(2) It represents a repetition of childhood conflicts
(3) It is considered a serious impediment to analysis
(4) It includes both transference symptoms and transference resistance

393. According to psychoanalytic dream theory, dreams can be described by which of the following statements?

(1) They often express transference wishes
(2) They are disguised and condensed expressions of unconscious mental content
(3) They have meaning in relation to the life of the dreamer
(4) They frequently involve the events of the preceding day

394. Psychoanalytic psychotherapies are characterized by a strong emphasis on the importance of which of the following?

(1) Unconscious motivation of behavior
(2) Precise descriptive diagnosis
(3) Concern with psychological defenses
(4) Phenomenology of symptoms

395. Violent behavior can be described by which of the following statements?

(1) It usually is committed by persons who have been exposed to violence in the past
(2) It can be lessened by individual and family psychotherapy
(3) It frequently is associated with alcohol intoxication
(4) Its occurrence can be predicted accurately by careful assessment of violence-prone persons

396. Normal grief reactions are characterized by which of the following statements?

(1) They typically begin with a state of emotional numbness or blunting
(2) They are usually worse if preceded by a period of anticipatory grief
(3) They are associated with increased rates of illness and death among bereaved persons
(4) The use of antidepressant medication effectively shortens the symptomatic period

397. Although the treatment of schizo-phrenia remains a controversial matter, current research focusing on methods of therapy suggests that

(1) intensive insight-oriented psycho-therapy is an effective treatment of acutely psychotic patients
(2) a maintenance neuroleptic drug regimen is effective in preventing recurrence of psychosis in many patients
(3) social and psychological treatments add little or nothing to effective pharmacological treatments
(4) phenothiazines are significantly more effective than placebo

398. A token economy involves which of the following therapeutic principles?

(1) Systematic desensitization
(2) Extinction
(3) Reciprocal inhibition
(4) Operant conditioning

399. The use of marital therapies gen-erally is contraindicated if

(1) one or both partners have secrets they do not want revealed
(2) one or both partners insist on a divorce
(3) one partner is anxious or fearful and refuses to participate
(4) one partner is psychotic

400. Transactional analysis can be de-scribed by which of the following state-ments?

(1) The concept of "lifescripts" is key
(2) It defines parent, adult, and child ego states
(3) It makes use of educational approaches
(4) It is an effective treatment of psychoses

401. Therapeutic measures used during brief psychotherapy can include

(1) crisis intervention
(2) use of psychotropic medication
(3) anxiety-suppressing techniques
(4) anxiety-provoking techniques

402. The Masters and Johnson treat-ment of sexually dysfunctional couples encourages

(1) careful identification of the dys-functional partner for focused indi-vidual treatment
(2) avoidance of sexual activity not specifically prescribed by the therapists
(3) early initiation of specialized tech-niques of genital intercourse
(4) direct discussion of sexual prefer-ences, dislikes, and fears

403. Important components of the psy-choanalytic interpretive process include

(1) transference
(2) dream interpretation
(3) an understanding of current patient conflicts
(4) timing

SUMMARY OF DIRECTIONS

A	B	C	D	E
1,2,3	1,3	2,4	4	All are
only	only	only	only	correct

404. Resistance that develops during analysis can be described by which of the following statements?

(1) It may be manifested by acting out
(2) It encompasses all the defensive operations presented by the patient
(3) It may be ego-alien or ego-syntonic
(4) It is easily recognized

405. Countertransference is described by which of the following statements?

(1) It concerns negative feelings developed by therapists toward their patients
(2) It concerns positive feelings developed by therapists toward their patients
(3) It can cause therapy to fail
(4) It can be of diagnostic and therapeutic use

406. Characteristics of the therapists in client-centered therapy should include

(1) genuineness (congruence)
(2) unconditional acceptance of the client
(3) empathic understanding of the client
(4) willingness to advise

407. In most sex therapies, treatment of premature ejaculation involves which of the following techniques?

(1) Sensate focus
(2) Stop-start technique
(3) Squeeze technique
(4) Use of anesthetic ointments

408. Behavior therapy employs which of the following techniques?

(1) Flooding
(2) Systematic desensitization
(3) Modeling
(4) Relaxation training

409. Psychodrama is a method of group therapy that can be described by which of the following statements?

(1) It is directly derived from psychoanalytic theory
(2) It makes use of an "auxiliary ego"
(3) It is especially suited for treating poorly motivated persons
(4) It involves the therapeutic use of role-playing and role-reversal

410. In contrast to adults in therapy, children in therapy tend to

(1) be highly motivated about their therapy
(2) develop early global transference reactions
(3) prefer internal resolution of problems
(4) show limited capacity for self-observation

411. "Working through" is characterized by

(1) identification of a defense
(2) understanding of the historical development of a defense
(3) discovery of the purpose of a defense
(4) development of new defenses

DIRECTIONS: The group of questions below consists of lettered headings followed by a set of numbered items. For each numbered item select the **one** lettered heading with which it is **most** closely associated. Each lettered heading may be used **once, more than once, or not at all.**

Questions 412–415

For each patient described, select the most appropriate therapeutic intervention.

   (A) Psychoanalysis
   (B) Brief individual psychotherapy
   (C) Community meeting
   (D) Behavior therapy
   (E) Family therapy

412. A young woman with no previous psychiatric history develops an incapacitating fear of driving after being involved in a minor automobile accident

413. A 40-year-old married man, a successful businessman with a satisfying family life, is preoccupied with thoughts of becoming involved with a younger woman. He has no prior psychiatric history and no other complaints

414. A 16-year-old girl begins acting out sexually. Her school performance deteriorates. These symptoms coincide with the outset of frequent arguments between her parents, who have been threatening marital separation

415. An intelligent 25-year-old single woman, who has a successful career, complains of multiple failed relationships with men, unhappiness, and a wish "to sort out my life." A previous experience in individual psychotherapy had been somewhat helpful

Psychotherapies
Answers

364. The answer is D. *(Michels, vol 1, chap 8, pp 6–7.)* Transference is a ubiquitous phenomenon, but it is especially prominent in psychoanalytic therapies because they are conducted so as to maximize its occurrence. The discovery of transference by Sigmund Freud was one of his most important contributions. Transference involves the patient's seeing and experiencing the present through "past-colored glasses," thereby making it possible to reconstruct the past and understand the origin of the patient's conflicts. While it certainly may color the patient's dreams, its predominant manifestations are in the interactions with the therapist or analyst in the course of treatment.

365. The answer is B. *(Talbott, pp 872–875.)* Cognitive psychotherapy is a directive and time-limited psychotherapy that aims to identify and eliminate negatively biased thinking so that the patient becomes more logical and reality based. It was originally developed as an intervention for nonpsychotic depressed patients. The therapist and patient, by "collaborative empiricism," identify the patient's irrational beliefs and illogical thinking pattern. They then devise methods so that the patient can test the validity of these beliefs and cognitions. The treatment is structured and behavioral, and it is not involved with dream interpretation or other vehicles for exploring the unconscious.

366. The answer is D. *(Michels, vol 1, chap 7, pp 6–7.)* There are a number of cognitive and motor performance tests that have been developed to evaluate or diagnose patients with neurological disorders and cerebral impairment. The Bender-Gestalt test of spacial relationships and constructional ability was one of the original and most widely used instruments. However, it cannot evaluate sufficiently the wide range of cognitive functions that may become impaired in organic brain syndromes. The Halstead-Reitan and the Luria-Nebraska tests involve sophisticated test batteries that evaluate a number of cognitive and psychomotor skills and may help to localize neurological impairment. The other listed tests may at times suggest the possibility of organicity, but that is not their major focus of inquiry.

367. The answer is B. *(Michels, vol 1, chap 31, pp 5–6.)* In the personality disorders, character traits are typically ego-syntonic. This means they usually cause the patient little personal distress, making motivation for change less likely. This is in contrast to neurotic symptoms, which are experienced as unwanted "foreign bodies.'' The patient's character traits often cause great distress to those who must live with them. Character traits are formed in response to developmental relationships and conflict, as are neurotic symptoms. They become part of the patient's style of living and relating to others.

368. The answer is A. *(Talbott, pp 878–882.)* Supportive psychotherapy is generally employed for crisis intervention, and with patients whose ego-deficits or life circumstance make other forms of therapy inappropriate or impractical. The therapist attempts to maintain a reality-based, problem-solving, concerned relationship that will augment the patient's ego-strengths and defenses. Commonly this will include giving advice, reassurance, and suggestion and assisting in reality testing. The treatment is not structured so as to maximize the likelihood of transference distortions as, for example, in psychoanalytic psychotherapy. Regression would not be encouraged, either in the transference or in general behavior.

369. The answer is A. *(Bassuk, pp 261–270. Michels, vol 1, chap 41, p 15.)* It is generally agreed that early intervention will help prevent stress-response syndromes from becoming chronic and will shorten the required treatment time. Brief psychotherapies, often dynamic in nature, are most commonly employed. Antidepressants are generally not indicated in the treatment of acute grief reactions. One must caution patients about continuing activities that require attention and concentration (e.g., driving, operating potentially dangerous machinery) during the acute phase, since these mental functions are often impaired. Crisis intervention may include helping the patient with preexisting conflicts that are associated with vulnerability, since one goal of treatment is to help the patient to be less vulnerable in the future to similar stressors.

370. The answer is D. *(Colarusso, pp 27–33. Talbott, pp 145–146.)* Erikson postulates that the life cycle consists of eight stages of ego development, commencing with birth and ending with death. The stages are based on the principle of epigenesis. Like the human embryo, personality development follows a predetermined sequence of steps that is governed by inner laws of development. Each developmental stage is characterized by a specific conflict during which opposing psychosocial attitudes vie for ascendancy. This creates a specific developmental crisis, the resolution of which allows each person to move on to the next developmental stage. Unlike Freud, who was primarily concerned with childhood psychosexual development, Erikson believes that personality develops throughout life. Generativity refers to central tasks of Erikson's stage of adulthood. These include caring for, and training, the next generation, betterment of society, and the production of ideas through one's work.

371. The answer is C. *(Talbott, pp 934-935.)* Masters and Johnson's therapy for anorgasmia is basically a behavioral approach to the treatment of sexual dysfunction, though some therapists include psychodynamic considerations. This is a couples-oriented approach, in which both partners participate from the beginning of treatment. In conjoint interviews they are encouraged to discover the nature of the problem, to understand each other's sexual experience, to dispel myths and inaccuracies about sex, and to become comfortable with sexual enjoyment. This may include encouraging solitary sexual pleasuring in which there is less anxiety provoked and then progressing to a graded series of exercises in which the couple becomes more comfortable with pleasuring each other. They are instructed not to have intercourse until late in the treatment, thereby removing a major source of anxiety regarding performance.

372. The answer is E. *(Kaplan, ed 4. pp 410–412.)* Criteria for the analyzability of a person's neurosis include all the following: the ability to test reality; a sense of trust in the therapist as well as in oneself to face unpleasant issues; the ability to tolerate dependence; the capacity to internalize experience; and the motivation to pursue an unknown course. Although the above qualities suggest the presence of a certain degree of maturity, analysis can be undertaken in adolescence.

373. The answer is D. *(Kaplan, ed 4. pp 410–412.)* Psychoanalysis is a commonly used treatment for persons who have long-standing neurotic problems or character disorders. These problems include conversion disorders, phobias, obsessive compulsive neuroses, and certain perversions. Generally, persons who are psychotic or addicted to drugs or alcohol have underlying pathology too severe to withstand the demands of analysis. There are, of course, exceptions.

374. The answer is D. *(Talbott, pp 868-869.)* Interpersonal psychotherapy is a brief treatment focusing on interpersonal problems and was developed for patients with nonpsychotic major depression. It is an individual psychotherapy aiming to improve communication and reality testing, clarify feeling states, and facilitate interpersonal skills. It is usually combined with antidepressant medication. While the treatment is based on psychodynamic theory, the focus is on current interpersonal events rather than intrapsychic issues.

375. The answer is C. *(Talbott, pp 856–860.)* Lateness is a characteristic resistance, which often has the goal of avoiding unpleasant or disturbing issues in therapy. If lateness occurs repeatedly during therapy, the therapist should explore the meaning of the behavior with the patient. Persistence on the part of the therapist, despite a myriad of excuses offered by the patient, often results in a precise determination of the reasons behind the lateness.

376. The answer is C. *(Kaplan, ed 4. pp 739–742.)* Therapists' attitudes toward the schizophrenic patient are a central aspect of therapeutic technique. If therapists feel they must rescue the schizophrenic patient, negative therapeutic reactions may result. Therapists should be more concerned with being of use to those patients. McGlashan has delineated several important aspects of therapists' attitudes toward schizophrenic patients. These include the importance of the therapist's consistency and availability, respect for the patient, valuing the patient's autonomy, an ability to focus on the patient's assets, tolerance for negative, bizarre, and incomprehensible behavior, and therapeutic optimism.

377. The answer is D. *(Kaplan, ed 4. pp 1403–1419.)* Many processes important to group therapy have been described. Cohesion is a fundamental process by which members develop a sense of belonging or loyalty. The group may draw on an individual's desire to "belong" when it exerts group pressure to initiate change in the individual. The group also provides a variety of models of behavior that group members may imitate. By universalization, a phenomenon common to groups, members learn that others have problems similar to their own. The goal is not to suppress individuality, but to help the patient understand how his or her unique individuality affects others, and vice versa.

378. The answer is A. *(Kaplan, ed 4. p 1414.)* Group therapy has been helpful in the treatment of patients who have a wide range of neurotic, psychotic, and personality disorders. Persons who have major mood disorders, however, are helped least by group therapy. Not only do severely depressed individuals, especially those who are suicidal, require more support and attention than is available in groups, but group therapy itself may aggravate symptoms of depression. Manic individuals tend to disrupt groups and usually are too restless to derive much benefit from group therapy. However, once their acute mania is controlled, they can profit from group treatment.

379. The answer is E (all). *(Michels, vol 2, chap 109, pp 4–11.)* Biofeedback usually employs instrumentation designed to provide the patient with visual or auditory feedback regarding physiological processes. For example, the electroencephalograph may be designed so as to emit a designated tone when alpha waves are achieved through relaxation. The electromyograph might be used to monitor activity in a specific group of muscles, with a visual or auditory signal that is proportional to the degree of relaxation achieved by the patient. Biofeedback has proved to be a useful adjunctive treatment in such conditions as migraine, hypertension, and chronic pain. In the case of headache due to muscle contraction, and for fecal incontinence due to sphincter incompetence or impaired ability to perceive rectal distention, it is often a treatment of choice.

380. The answer is C (2, 4). *(Kaplan, ed 4. pp 1389–1391.)* Hypnosis is best described as a state of intense, focused alertness with a constriction of peripheral awareness. The EEG during a hypnotic trance shows that the brain is experiencing resting arousal. The use of hypnosis by healers dates back centuries. Early in his studies of the unconscious, Freud employed hypnosis to help patients reexperience and abreact early life trauma. He soon abandoned it in favor of analysis of the transference. It is believed that about two-thirds of psychiatric outpatient populations are hypnotizable.

381. The answer is E (all). *(Kaplan, ed 4. pp 1432–1434.)* Cognitive theory relates the development of psychiatric symptoms and syndromes to habitual errors in thinking (cognition). The depressed person is viewed as one whose symptoms and affects are the logical outcome of negative cognitive patterns. Self, experience, and future are viewed through "negative colored glasses." Cognitions are developed early in life and may be activated by a life situation or stress.

382. The answer is E (all). *(Michels, vol 1, chap 33, pp 11–13.)* The most common treatment for agoraphobia combines drugs with behavior modification or psychotherapy or both. Drugs that have proved particularly useful are the tricyclic antidepressants, the monoamine oxidase (MAO) inhibitors, and alprazolam. Antidepressant medication helps to block the occurrence of spontaneous panic attacks, and alprazolam may also have an effect on anticipatory anxiety. Psychotherapy, often supportive in nature, and behavioral techniques are used to help the patient reenter phobic situations and decondition their anticipatory anxiety and avoidance.

383. The answer is D (4). *(Michels, vol 1, chap 45, pp 4–7.)* DSM III-R reflects the current view of most mental health professionals that homosexuality per se should not be regarded as a form of psychopathology. It is not listed as a mental disorder on axis I or II. The term *ego dystonic homosexuality* is sometimes used to describe those who have unwanted homosexual arousal and who wish to increase heterosexual arousal. There are more similarities than differences between homosexuals and heterosexuals with regard to most categories of psychopathology. There are many people who feel an inner identity as a homosexual, but live an exclusively heterosexual life with regard to behavior. There are also many people whose inner identity is heterosexual, but who have homosexual fantasies that may or may not be reflective of sexual or nonsexual conflict.

384. The answer is E (all). *(Kaplan, ed 4. pp 1093–1096.)* Increasing attention is now being paid to adults who were victims of childhood incest. These patients, usually women, complain of a number of psychiatric symptoms, including depression, anxiety, sexual dysfunction (promiscuity, orgasmic dysfunction), guilt, low self-esteem, drug and alcohol abuse, marital problems, and somatization. The risk of incest and of physical and emotional abuse is increased for their children. Many of the former victims of childhood sexual abuse do not immediately disclose this history. For treatment to be successful, it must deal with the abuse and its effects.

385. The answer is C (2, 4). *(Michels, vol 2, chap 81, pp 1–3; vol 3, chap 45, pp 8–9.)* Placebos are pharmacologically inert substances that the user believes are potent drugs. Placebos have been shown to be effective in relieving a variety of neurotic symptoms, including anxiety and depression. They often produce side effects, such as weakness, headache, and gastrointestinal symptoms. Placebo effects are influenced strongly by the attitudes and expectations of both physician and patient. Primary schizophrenic symptoms and endogenous depression do not respond to placebos.

386. The answer is D (4). *(Kaplan, ed 4. pp 1389–1397.)* Hypnosis can be used to increase a person's control of symptoms and to uncover repressed material. Hypnosis is a state of resting alertness and is not related to sleep. Persons with severe psychopathology are generally less hypnotizable than other persons. The "eye roll" sign and other clinical indices have been found to correlate with susceptibility to hypnosis. Like all persons in a therapeutic setting, hypnotic subjects can be abused or exploited; however, the hypnotic state is not inherently dangerous.

387. The answer is C (2, 4). *(Kaplan, ed 4. p 713.)* Psychotherapy alone has been found to be less effective than drug treatment alone. Drug treatment in conjunction with psychotherapy appears to provide the best protection against recurrence of psychotic symptoms. Psychotherapy may have an adverse effect on some withdrawn schizophrenic patients.

388. The answer is A (1, 2, 3). *(Kaplan, ed 4. pp 1366–1367.)* Systematic desensitization is a technique of behavior therapy in which a patient in a state of profound muscular relaxation is asked to imagine specific anxiety-provoking scenes, which have been arranged in a hierarchical sequence beginning with the least provocative. When a subject is able to imagine a scene without becoming anxious, the therapist presents the next, more anxiety-provoking scene in the hierarchy. Systematic desensitization has been used in treating patients who have phobias, obsessive compulsive behaviors, and certain sexual problems.

389. The answer is E (all). *(Michels, vol 1, chap 71, pp 11–17.)* The proper management of the suicidal patient is one of the most difficult tasks facing psychiatric clinicians. Ensuring the patient's safety is the most immediate problem to be dealt with. Continuous observation of the patient, removal of harmful objects, and education of hospital staff regarding suicidal behavior are all geared to provide for the optimal safety and treatment of the suicidal patient. Bathrooms are the most common area in which inpatient suicides occur, and hanging is the most common method. Thus, bathrooms must be very carefully designed, and actively suicidal patients should be accompanied to the bathroom. The accompanying attendant may remain out of sight but should have verbal contact with the patient every few minutes.

390. The answer is B (1, 3). *(Kaplan, ed 4. pp 1438–1443.)* Existential psychotherapy departs from traditional psychiatry in that emphasis is placed on a person's own sense of the meaning of his or her life rather than on psychopathology and past development. Spiritual values also are important in existential psychotherapy. Exponents of this view suggest that each individual determines his or her own nature by a constant act of self-definition for which the individual is solely responsible.

391. The answer is E (all). *(Kaplan, ed 4. pp 1582–1586.)* Psychiatric patients in day hospital programs spend their daytime hours in a hospital setting but go home during evenings and weekends. Day hospital programs may provide a useful transition from inpatient care for partially stabilized patients who are not yet fully ready to return to the community. For selected patients, a day hospital may be a more effective treatment setting than an inpatient facility. Similarly, a day hospital may be more effective than regular outpatient treatment for certain chronically psychotic patients and may be a valuable alternative to nursing home placement for many older persons.

392. The answer is C (2, 4). *(Kaplan, ed 4. pp 1342–1343.)* Development of a transference neurosis marks the middle phase of analysis in which the analysand relives the conflicts of the infantile neurosis. In this middle period, the patient becomes extremely concerned with matters relating to the analysis; other problems seem to pale by comparison. Transference neurosis, which includes both transference symptoms and transference resistance, was originally thought to impede analysis; however, analysts now regard it as an effective means of permitting first-hand observation of childhood conflicts.

393. The answer is E (all). *(Kaplan, ed 4. p 1347.)* Psychoanalysis makes frequent use of dream analysis as a therapeutic tool to explore a person's unconscious thoughts. Psychoanalytic dream theory views dreams as distorted, disguised, and condensed expressions of the dreamer's unconscious wishes that permit unacceptable wishes to be fulfilled in the form of "hallucinations" during sleep. Thus, dreams contain valuable, though disguised, clues to the unconscious mental life of the dreamer. Recent experience often appears in dreams; this "day residue" is thought to be relatively neutral material used to construct the dream, the symbolic and thematic content of which is unconsciously motivated. Dreams often express the unfolding of the transference neurosis.

394. The answer is B (1, 3). *(Kaplan, ed 4. pp 1353–1361.)* A variety of different psychotherapies are based on psychodynamic principles. These therapies include psychoanalysis, psychoanalytic psychotherapy, relationship therapy, some supportive therapies, and others. Psychodynamic principles focus on the forces and motivations underlying human thought, feeling, and action. In particular, they are concerned with unconscious motivation in psychopathological experience and behavior. This concern is reflected in part in the attention dynamic therapists give to the resistances and psychological defenses of their patients. In contrast to dynamic psychiatry, descriptive psychiatry emphasizes precise diagnosis and careful observation of symptoms and behavior.

395. The answer is A (1, 2, 3). *(Michels, vol 2, chap 95, pp 7–8; vol 3, chap 32, pp 7–8.)* Violent behavior, especially when impulsive or irrational, frequently is associated with mental illness. Violent persons typically have been exposed to a culture that endorses violence or were raised in a family in which violence was common. Intoxicated persons frequently exaggerate the hostile intentions of others and misjudge the consequences of violent acts. Repeated studies have demonstrated a high correlation between alcohol intoxication and violence. Individual and family treatment can help to resolve the conflicts and alter the patterns of behavior that can lead to violent outbursts. Although previous episodes of violent behavior and other factors increase the likelihood of violence, the occurrence of violent behavior is very difficult to predict. Psychiatrists are often unable to predict accurately whether a person is likely to commit violent acts and have tended to overpredict violence markedly.

396. The answer is B (1, 3). *(Kaplan, ed 4. pp 1286–1293.)* Normal grief reactions typically begin with a period of shock and numbness, followed by a period of yearning and protest. The next, final phase is one of apathy and aimlessness. Anticipatory grief may reduce the severity of grief reactions in some instances. Bereaved persons have an increased incidence of both physical and emotional illness, as well as a higher mortality. They may benefit from the judicious use of sedatives and antianxiety agents, but pharmacological suppression of the symptoms of mourning can be harmful.

397. The answer is C (2, 4). *(Kaplan, ed 4. pp 713, 716–720.)* Recent research suggests that neuroleptic medications are effective in the treatment of acute psychosis and important in the prevention of relapse for a significant minority of schizophrenic patients. In double-blind studies, neuroleptics repeatedly have been shown to be more effective than placebo. Social and psychological interventions add significantly to the overall effectiveness of comprehensive treatment of schizophrenic patients. There is little evidence to support the notion that intensive insight-oriented therapy is effective in the treatment of acute psychotic symptoms.

398. The answer is C (2, 4). *(Kaplan, ed 4. pp 1369–1370.)* A token economy is an example of a treatment based on principles of operant conditioning. Positive reinforcement is used to reward desired behavior. Because inappropriate behavior is not rewarded, its frequency decreases; this process is known as extinction. Desensitization and reciprocal inhibition are principles of classical conditioning, not operant conditioning.

399. The answer is A (1, 2, 3). *(Kaplan, ed 4. pp 1444–1445.)* Contraindications to marital therapy include the refusal of a partner to participate, the existence of secrets that cannot be revealed, and the insistence of one or both partners on the need for a divorce. Psychosis in one or both partners need not be a contraindication to marital therapy. In fact, marital therapy may be the treatment of choice in selected cases of psychosis precipitated by marital discord.

400. The answer is A (1, 2, 3). *(Kaplan, ed 4. pp 1452–1453.)* Transactional analysis, which was developed by Eric Berne, is basically an outgrowth of psychoanalytic theory. The parent, adult, and child ego states are in many ways similar to the classic division of superego, ego, and id. Transactions are interactions between ego states. The theory behind transactional analysis is that people choose their "lifescripts" as children and that this choice influences their relationships throughout their lives. The approach of the therapist often is educational, making use of lectures and related techniques. Transactional analysis has generally been used to treat minimally disturbed patients, not those who are severely ill or psychotic.

401. The answer is E (all). *(Kaplan, ed 4. pp 1361–1363.)* Brief psychotherapies can be divided into two basic treatment types: anxiety-suppressive (or supportive) treatments and anxiety-provoking treatments. Anxiety-suppressive techniques include reassurance, active intervention by the therapist, environmental manipulation, brief hospitalization, and the use of psychotropic medication. Anxiety-provoking techniques involve focused interpretive work with carefully selected, highly motivated patients. Patients in crisis may be treated with either technique, depending on the severity of their problems and their level of motivation.

402. The answer is C (2, 4). *(Kaplan, ed 4. pp 1087–1088.)* As described by William Masters and Virginia Johnson, the techniques involved in the treatment of sexual dysfunction draw on the principles of education, behavior therapy, and couples therapy. Treatment of the couple rather than of one partner is emphasized. Educational aspects of the treatment are designed primarily to correct misinformation. Each partner is encouraged to voice fears, preferences, and dislikes in order to enlighten the other and clarify sexual attitudes. The treatment of common disorders, such as impotence, premature ejaculation, and vaginismus, involves the use of a sequence of carefully structured exercises designed to minimize anxiety and facilitate pleasurable responses. Genital intercourse is avoided until the couple has mastered less-threatening exercises; similarly, while treatment is in progress, the couple is advised to avoid sexual activity not prescribed by the therapists.

403. The answer is E (all). *(Kaplan, ed 4. pp 414–417.)* In the interpretive process, the analyst gives meaning to those psychological events that are incomprehensible to the patient. Clarification of the patient's ambiguous statements is the key to interpretation. The interpretive process makes use of transference and dream interpretation and relates current patient conflicts to factors in the patient's past. Timing is critical; generally, an interpretation should be presented just before patients understand it on their own.

404. The answer is A (1, 2, 3). *(Kaplan, ed 4. pp 414–415.)* Resistance refers to the behavior a patient presents when defending against impulses uncovered in therapy. All the defensive operations that a patient employs are included in resistance. Resistances may be either ego-syntonic or ego-alien, and some, including acting out, may be hard to recognize.

405. The answer is E (all). *(Kaplan, ed 4. pp 1345–1347.)* Countertransference refers to the development by a therapist of feelings and attitudes toward a patient. These feelings, which can be both positive and negative, are the combined result of the patient's impact on the mind and personality of the therapist. Therapists can make use of their emotional reactions to their patients, helping to clarify diagnostic and therapeutic problems. However, if unrecognized or unchecked, countertransference can cause therapy to fail.

406. The answer is A (1, 2, 3). *(Kaplan, ed 4. pp 1374–1384.)* The attitudes of therapists in client-centered therapy should include those of genuineness and sincerity. Therapy should be based on the therapists' unconditional acceptance of and deep regard for their clients. Although therapists should demonstrate an empathic understanding of their clients, they should keep advice to a minimum and scrupulously avoid meddling in or manipulating clients' affairs.

407. The answer is A (1, 2, 3). *(Kaplan, ed 4. pp 1087–1088.)* The success rate in the treatment of premature ejaculation tends to be quite high. The treatment involves both partners and begins with sensate focus, a series of exercises designed to increase awareness of pleasurable touch, sound, and sight. The "squeeze technique" is an exercise in which the penis is stimulated to the first sensations of impending orgasm and then strongly squeezed at the coronal ridge, causing partial loss of erection. The stop-start technique consists of stimulating the man to a point just short of inevitable orgasm; at that point, stimulation is halted until the sensation of impending orgasm disappears. The use of anesthetic ointments has proved unsatisfactory in the treatment of premature ejaculation.

408. The answer is E (all). *(Michels, vol 2, chap 77, pp 7–15.)* Behavior therapy is based on the work of Ivan Pavlov, Joseph Wolpe, and others. It focuses on observable patient behavior, rather than on inferred mental states. The principles of conditioning and learning are important theoretical foundations of this approach. Systematic desensitization, a key technique in behavior therapy, permits a patient to overcome anxiety by gradually confronting an anxiety-provoking stimulus in a relaxed state. Flooding is a technique in which a patient directly confronts an intensely anxiety-provoking situation, is "flooded" with anxiety, and remains in this situation until calm and able to experience a sense of mastery. Modeling involves the overcoming of anxiety by observing and imitating a model who is free of that symptom. Relaxation training is the most common tool used by behavior therapists as an adjunct to other techniques, such as desensitization.

409. The answer is C (2, 4). (*Kaplan, ed 4. pp 1423–1427.*) Psychodrama is a form of group psychotherapy developed by Jacob L. Moreno. Its development was contemporary with but separate from that of psychoanalysis. The degree of self-exposure required in psychodrama makes it most suitable for treating highly motivated persons. In psychodramatic treatment, the patient becomes the "protagonist" in the drama; another group member becomes the "auxiliary ego" and plays the role of a person or an element important to the protagonist. Role-playing and role-reversal are techniques commonly employed in psychodrama.

410. The answer is C (2, 4). (*Kaplan, ed 4. p 1776.*) In dealing with internal conflicts, children tend to choose alloplastic or externally manipulated adaptations rather than internal modifications. In addition, they have a limited capacity for self-observation. Although global transference reactions occur early in the course of therapy, the value of subsequent transference reactions is limited. Because children generally are taken to treatment by a parent or teacher, their motivation for treatment usually is less than that exhibited by adults.

411. The answer is E (all). (*Kaplan, ed 4. p 1344.*) The process of working through begins with the recognition by analyst and patient of the patient's defensive maneuvers. The analyst then demonstrates that the defense is historically determined and is used to evade some drive and prevent this drive from becoming conscious. The process of working through must be repeated many times, because the patient soon presents new variations of the defensive behavior. This process seems to speed up, however, as more of these interpretative confrontations occur.

412. The answer is D. (*Kaplan, ed 4. p 1367.*) Systematic desensitization, which is a form of behavior therapy, is the most appropriate treatment for this woman. Systematic desensitization is used to treat classic phobias, but this technique as well as other forms of behavior therapy may also be of benefit in the treatment of other psychiatric disorders. It would be expected to be a good choice of treatment since the phobia appears to be unassociated with other complicating psychiatric problems.

413. The answer is B. (*Kaplan, ed 4. pp 1361–1362.*) Patient selection is an important aspect of brief psychotherapy. Utilizing psychoanalytic principles, the clinician attempts to select patients who are above average in intelligence, motivated, and able to think psychologically. Having a focused chief complaint, e.g., this man's interest in a younger woman, is also crucial. Given this man's good work history, family life, lack of previous psychotherapy, and focused complaint, brief psychotherapy is a suitable treatment. Were it to uncover other, significant problem areas, then a longer term therapy might be indicated.

414. The answer is E. *(Kaplan, ed 4. pp 1427–1432.)* Family therapy is a treatment of choice because this girl's symptomatic behavior appears to be linked to her parents' marital difficulties. Individual treatment, which would address the girl's symptoms, would not alter the marital or family problems, nor would it allow the parents to explore the impact of their daughter's symptoms on the marital relationship.

415. The answer is A. *(Kaplan, ed 4. p 1357.)* This woman is likely to be an appropriate candidate for psychoanalysis. She describes long-standing problems in heterosexual relationships. These are likely to be due to unconscious conflicts. In addition, she is unhappy with her life. Because previous psychotherapy helped but did not stop her symptoms, assessment for psychoanalysis is a reasonable therapeutic intervention.

Psychopharmacology and Other Therapies

DIRECTIONS: Each question below contains five suggested responses. Select the **one best** response to each question.

416. Which of the following statements regarding benzodiazepine receptors is true?

(A) To date, there has been only one type of benzodiazepine receptor identified
(B) Benzodiazepine receptors are all presynaptic
(C) Benzodiazepine receptors are measured using oxazepam
(D) Benzodiazepine receptors are all affected by gamma-aminobutyric acid (GABA)
(E) Benzodiazepine receptors have little stereospecificity

417. All the following are capable of increasing plasma levels of lithium EXCEPT

(A) thiazide diuretics
(B) indomethacin
(C) fasting and low-salt diets
(D) phenylbutazone
(E) high intake of coffee

418. All the following statements about carbamazepine are true EXCEPT

(A) it is used in the treatment of mania
(B) it is used in the treatment of severe anxiety disorders
(C) it may cause fatal aplastic anemia
(D) it is potentially hepatotoxic
(E) it has mild anticholinergic activity

419. All the following statements about electroconvulsive therapy (ECT) are true EXCEPT

(A) the principal indication is for the treatment of severe depression
(B) it may be particularly effective in patients with delusional depression
(C) it may be of benefit in the treatment of manic excitement
(D) it is a procedure with a relatively high mortality
(E) it may be associated with impairment of memory

Questions 420–422

A 29-year-old woman is brought into the hospital by her husband after having charged her credit card to the limit while buying 40 pairs of identical shoes. Her husband reports she has not slept in 2 days and paces the house all night. Her speech is pressured and its content difficult to follow. Two weeks earlier she had been extremely depressed. The diagnosis of bipolar disorder, manic, is made.

420. Before starting the patient on lithium, all the following tests should be done EXCEPT

(A) BUN and creatinine
(B) chest x-ray
(C) thyroid panel
(D) ECG
(E) pregnancy test

421. The initial daily dosage of lithium should be tested at

(A) 150 mg
(B) 300 mg
(C) 600 mg
(D) 1200 mg
(E) 1800 mg

422. Therapeutic lithium levels are

(A) 0.4 to 0.8 mg%
(B) 0.8 to 1.5 mg%
(C) 0.2 to 0.6 mEq/L
(D) 0.8 to 1.2 mEq/L
(E) 1 to 1.5 mEq/g

423. A double-blind crossover drug study means

(A) the subject does not know whether he or she is getting drug or placebo during the study and is not told after completion of the study
(B) the researcher does not know if the subject is getting drug or placebo and is not told after completion of the study
(C) the subject is not told what he or she is taking and is switched from drug to placebo in mid-study
(D) neither the patient nor the researcher knows whether drug or placebo is being used, and a switch is made in mid-study
(E) none of the above

424. The half-life of a drug refers to

(A) how long the drug will last unused
(B) how long it takes to produce the drug
(C) how long the drug will remain at least one-half active
(D) how long it will take to metabolize one-half the drug
(E) the temperature a drug must be kept at to keep it from losing half its potency

425. Which of the following antipsychotics is the most potent?

(A) Chlorpromazine (Thorazine)
(B) Thiothixene (Navane)
(C) Trifluoperazine (Stelazine)
(D) Haloperidol (Haldol)
(E) Thioridazine (Mellaril)

426. The tricyclic antidepressants are effective because of their ability to

(A) block postsynaptic dopamine receptors
(B) inhibit dopamine release
(C) inhibit the reuptake of dopamine
(D) inhibit the reuptake of serotonin and norepinephrine
(E) inhibit the release of monoamine oxidase

427. Side effects seen with tricyclic antidepressants include all the following EXCEPT

(A) dry mouth
(B) urinary retention
(C) involuntary muscle movements
(D) orthostatic hypotension
(E) constipation

428. Which of the following psychotropic medications can produce psychotic delusions, manic elation, or disorientation in some patients?

(A) Diazepam
(B) Lithium
(C) Amitriptyline
(D) Chlorpromazine
(E) Phenytoin

429. A man who has agitated depression is started on the following medications (in daily dosages): imipramine, 150 mg; perphenazine, 32 mg; and benztropine mesylate (Cogentin), 2 mg. One week later, his wife reports that he has been unusually forgetful during the last 4 days and that last night he awoke unusually confused about where he was. On physical examination, the man appears slightly flushed, his skin and palms are dry, and his heart rate is fast. He is slow to remember the date and has trouble concentrating. He showed none of these symptoms during his appointment last week. The diagnosis is

(A) extrapyramidal syndrome
(B) neuroleptic syndrome
(C) schizophreniform psychosis
(D) toxic brain syndrome
(E) cerebrovascular accident

430. Which of the following drugs has shown the greatest efficacy in treating obsessive compulsive disorder?

(A) Chlordiazepoxide
(B) Clomipramine
(C) Perphenazine
(D) Chlorpromazine
(E) Lithium

431. Which of the following statements best describes the development of tolerance during chronic administration of benzodiazepines (e.g., diazepam)?

(A) No tolerance develops
(B) Tolerance develops to the sedating effect but not to the antianxiety effect
(C) Tolerance develops to the antianxiety effect but not to the sedating effect
(D) Tolerance develops to both the sedating and antianxiety effects
(E) Tolerance develops only in persons who have addictive personalities

432. The antimanic effect of lithium usually is observed within

(A) 2 days
(B) 5 days
(C) 10 days
(D) 15 days
(E) 21 days

433. The duration of action of a single dose of fluphenazine decanoate (Prolixin Decanoate) is

(A) 30 minutes
(B) 2 hours
(C) 3 days
(D) 2 weeks
(E) 2 months

434. The minimum daily dosage of chlorpromazine (Thorazine) needed to produce a therapeutic effect in most psychotic persons is

(A) 10 mg
(B) 50 mg
(C) 300 mg
(D) 800 mg
(E) 1500 mg

435. The mechanism of action of antipsychotic drugs currently is believed to involve blockade at receptor sites for which of the following compounds?

(A) Histamine
(B) Dopamine
(C) Acetylcholine
(D) Epinephrine
(E) Gamma-aminobutyric acid

436. Which of the following drugs has the most pronounced anticholinergic effects?

(A) Amitriptyline
(B) Perphenazine
(C) Chlordiazepoxide
(D) Lithium
(E) Desipramine

437. Severe reactions and death have been reported in persons who had been taking an MAO inhibitor and then were given

(A) chlorpromazine
(B) diazepam
(C) lithium
(D) imipramine
(E) phenobarbital

438. Which of the following drugs is LEAST sedating?

(A) Chlorpromazine
(B) Imipramine
(C) Diazepam
(D) Lithium
(E) Haloperidol

439. During a 2-month period, a 72-year-old woman who has senile dementia becomes increasingly withdrawn, shows little interest in food, has trouble sleeping, and appears to become more severely demented. Her medical status is unchanged. Which of the following courses of treatment would be the most reasonable?

(A) Bedtime sedation to improve sleep
(B) Diazepam, 5 mg three times daily
(C) A trial of tricyclic antidepressants
(D) A trial of perphenazine, 4 mg three times daily
(E) None of the above, because her condition is untreatable

440. The first few weeks of methylphenidate treatment for children who have attention deficit disorder may be marked by improvements in all the following areas EXCEPT

(A) attention span
(B) scores on achievement tests
(C) tolerance to frustration
(D) responsiveness to family and friends
(E) performance in school

441. In the treatment of persons in alcoholic withdrawal, chlordiazepoxide (Librium) commonly is used in daily dosages as high as

(A) 50 mg
(B) 100 mg
(C) 400 mg
(D) 1000 mg
(E) 2000 mg

442. The serum level of lithium at which therapeutic benefit levels off and side effects increase usually is considered to be

(A) 0.5 mEq/L
(B) 1.0 mEq/L
(C) 1.5 mEq/L
(D) 2.0 mEq/L
(E) 3.0 mEq/L

443. Physicians caring for persons who have taken an overdose of tricyclic antidepressants should pay special attention to which of the following clinical indicators?

(A) Renal output
(B) Cardiac rhythm
(C) Serum levels of bilirubin
(D) Bowel sounds
(E) Serum levels of glutamic oxaloacetic transaminase (SGOT)

444. Clinical response to an adequate dosage of tricyclic antidepressants typically occurs how long after initiation of treatment?

(A) 4 to 8 hours
(B) 1 to 3 days
(C) 3 to 7 days
(D) 5 to 10 days
(E) 7 to 21 days

445. In the order presented, the medications thioridazine (Mellaril), chlorpromazine, perphenazine (Trilafon), and haloperidol (Haldol) are characterized by

(A) increasing hypotensive effects but decreasing sedative effects
(B) increasing hypotensive effects but decreasing extrapyramidal effects
(C) increasing extrapyramidal effects but decreasing anticholinergic effects
(D) increasing anticholinergic effects but decreasing hypotensive effects
(E) increasing sedative effects but decreasing anticholinergic effects

446. The various antipsychotic drugs currently in use are all about equal in terms of

(A) cost
(B) side effects
(C) milligram potency
(D) antipsychotic effectiveness
(E) antiemetic effectiveness

447. The daily dosage range of imipramine that is effective for the treatment of most depressed adults is

(A) 2 to 25 mg
(B) 10 to 100 mg
(C) 25 to 150 mg
(D) 75 to 300 mg
(E) 200 to 800 mg

448. Tricyclic antidepressants block the action of which of the following drugs?

(A) Chlorpromazine
(B) Guanethidine (Ismelin)
(C) Diazepam (Valium)
(D) Phenytoin (Dilantin)
(E) Quinidine

449. Gilles de la Tourette's syndrome is a childhood disorder that often begins with facial tics and progresses to multiple tics, grimacing, and spasmodic utterances. Patients with this disease have been treated successfully with

(A) chlordiazepoxide
(B) haloperidol
(C) methylphenidate (Ritalin)
(D) tranylcypromine (Parnate)
(E) protriptyline (Vivactil)

450. In elderly persons, increased confusion and paradoxical agitation are most likely to be associated with administration of which of the following sleep-inducing medications?

(A) Secobarbital (Seconal)
(B) Flurazepam (Dalmane)
(C) Chloral hydrate
(D) Chlorpromazine
(E) Amitriptyline

451. Epinephrine is contraindicated for the treatment of hypotension in persons taking

(A) diazepam
(B) lithium
(C) amitriptyline
(D) imipramine
(E) chlorpromazine

DIRECTIONS: Each question below contains four suggested responses of which **one or more** is correct. Select

A	if	**1, 2, and 3**	are correct
B	if	**1 and 3**	are correct
C	if	**2 and 4**	are correct
D	if	**4**	is correct
E	if	**1, 2, 3, and 4**	are correct

452. Seasonal depression is often treated by

(1) antidepressant medication
(2) neuroleptic medication
(3) light (phototherapy)
(4) carbamazepine

453. A woman is being treated with medication for her schizophrenia. Which of the following medications might be effective in controlling her psychotic symptoms?

(1) Haloperidol (Haldol)
(2) Chlorpromazine (Thorazine)
(3) Thiothixene (Navane)
(4) Lithium

454. Medications produced from opium include

(1) morphine
(2) thorazine
(3) codeine
(4) diazepam

Questions 455–457

An acutely psychotic woman is being treated with chlorpromazine, 400 mg daily. After 7 days, the woman's psychotic symptoms have not abated.

455. During the first few weeks of treatment the woman may develop extrapyramidal symptoms. These may take the form of

(1) an acute dystonic reaction
(2) akathisia
(3) a parkinsonian syndrome
(4) tardive dyskinesia

456. The woman begins to complain of dry mouth, blurred vision, and constipation. As a result, her physician should

(1) consider that her psychosis may be getting worse
(2) adjust the chlorpromazine dosage
(3) administer an anticholinergic drug
(4) ask her if she has difficulty initiating urination

457. A week after initiation of treatment, physical examination of the woman reveals cogwheel rigidity and resting tremor. Her physician also might expect to find which of the following?

(1) Intermittent euphoria
(2) Hypokinesia
(3) Corneal opacities
(4) Micrographia

458. The clinical application of plasma levels of antipsychotics

(1) enables titration of dosage to achieve optimal clinical effect
(2) is affected by the presence of active metabolites of antipsychotic drugs
(3) permits dosage adjustment to minimize extrapyramidal symptoms
(4) is limited by the poor correlation between drug level and clinical response

459. Benzodiazepines, such as diazepam, have some degree of cross-tolerance and cross-dependence with which of the following drugs?

(1) Alcohol
(2) Narcotic analgesics
(3) Barbiturates
(4) Phenothiazines

460. The clinical effectiveness of benzodiazepine medications can be described by which of the following statements?

(1) Meprobamate (Miltown, Equanil) shows a greater superiority over placebo in reducing anxiety than is shown by benzodiazepines
(2) Benzodiazepines are as effective in treating anxiety secondary to an affective disorder or schizophrenia as they are in treating simple anxiety
(3) Benzodiazepines are clearly superior to placebo in reducing acute anxiety
(4) Benzodiazepines are clearly superior to placebo in reducing chronic anxiety

461. Antidepressant drugs belonging to the tricyclic class include

(1) protriptyline
(2) maprotiline
(3) doxepin
(4) trazodone

462. Side effects that are relatively common during the first few days of lithium therapy include

(1) nausea and diarrhea
(2) blurred vision
(3) hand tremor
(4) masked facies

463. Endocrine effects of the phenothiazines include

(1) increased secretion of growth hormone
(2) galactorrhea
(3) weight loss
(4) amenorrhea

464. If a patient has been on pheno-thiazine therapy for several months, the abrupt withdrawal of the medication may lead to

(1) an acute craving for the drug
(2) muscular discomfort
(3) convulsions
(4) insomnia

465. Measures aimed at minimizing the long-term risks of tardive dyskine-sia associated with antipsychotic drug use include

(1) careful observation for early detec-tion of signs of tardive dyskinesia
(2) restriction of the chronic adminis-tration of antipsychotic drugs to those persons with psychosis or chronic anxiety
(3) discontinuation of antipsychotic drugs when signs of tardive dyski-nesia are detected
(4) prophylactic use of anticholinergic drugs in persons who have shown parkinsonian signs

466. Diazepam can be described by which of the following statements?

(1) Its administration is the preferred treatment of persons in status epi-lepticus
(2) It is a better muscle relaxant than is placebo
(3) It can eliminate stage-4 sleep
(4) It is not useful as a hypnotic agent

467. Lithium is clearly effective in the treatment of which of the following disorders?

(1) Schizophrenic psychosis
(2) Major depression
(3) Anxiety
(4) Mania

468. The use of lithium is contraindi-cated in the presence of which of the following factors?

(1) Salt-free diet
(2) Reduced hepatic function
(3) Very low creatinine clearance
(4) Concurrent use of an antidepres-sant agent

469. Common side effects of tricyclic antidepressants include

(1) postural hypotension
(2) bradycardia
(3) loss of the accommodation reflex
(4) diarrhea

470. Clinical actions of tricyclic anti-depressant drugs include which of the following?

(1) Depression of mood in manic per-sons
(2) Elevation of mood in normal per-sons
(3) Elevation of mood in demoralized persons
(4) Reduction of depression in persons who have primary depressive ill-ness

SUMMARY OF DIRECTIONS

A	B	C	D	E
1,2,3 only	1,3 only	2,4 only	4 only	All are correct

471. The action of reserpine has had an important influence on the development of the biogenic amine hypothesis of depression, because the drug can

(1) block reuptake of norepinephrine
(2) deplete nerve endings of norepinephrine and serotonin
(3) reduce blood pressure
(4) produce depression in humans

472. Imipramine has been demonstrated to be effective in the treatment of patients who have which of the following disorders?

(1) Mania
(2) Panic disorder
(3) Psychosis
(4) Obsessive compulsive personality disorder

473. Early central nervous system signs of lithium toxicity include

(1) seizures
(2) ataxia
(3) hyperreflexia
(4) dysarthria

474. A person taking a phenothiazine medication is likely to develop tolerance to which of the following effects of the drug?

(1) Sedation
(2) Lightheadedness
(3) Extrapyramidal reactions
(4) Antipsychotic actions

475. Major determinants of serious adverse effects in depressed patients receiving tricyclic antidepressants include

(1) elevated plasma levels of the drugs
(2) concurrent treatment with antipsychotic drugs
(3) concurrent treatment with non-psychotropic drugs
(4) advanced age

476. Correct statements regarding tardive dyskinesia include which of the following?

(1) It can be irreversible
(2) It can be life-threatening
(3) It commonly affects movements of the mouth and tongue
(4) It develops as a result of acute neuroleptic toxicity

Psychopharmacology and Other Therapies

Answers

416. The answer is D. *(Michels, vol 3, chap 50, p 9.)* Recent research has identified selective receptor-binding assays for benzodiazepines, having found H^3-diazepam binding sites in brain tissues. These binding sites exhibit stereospecificity and are divided into two types. Type I is anxiolytic and anticonvulsant without being sedating. These sites are found postsynaptically and are primarily in the cerebellum and cortex. Type II is presynaptic, is found mostly in the hippocampus, striatum, and brainstem, and causes sedation. Both types are affected by GABA.

417. The answer is E. *(Schatzberg, pp 123–124.)* When a patient is stabilized on lithium, and a thiazide diuretic is added in ignorance, the lithium level can double or reach toxicity. Low-salt diets and fasting can also decrease excretion of lithium, thereby increasing plasma levels. Indomethacin and phenylbutazone (nonsteroidal anti-inflammatory agents) have been reported to significantly decrease excretion of lithium. Clinicians should be alert to the possibility of a high intake of coffee interfering with achieving therapeutic levels of lithium.

418. The answer is B. *(Talbott, pp 827–828.)* Carbamazepine has been found to be effective in the treatment of acute manic episodes, as well as in the prophylactic treatment of mania. It is not used in the treatment of anxiety disorders. One problem with the use of this drug relates to its potential for hepatotoxicity and hematologic toxicity, including aplastic anemia. Since the drug has mild anticholinergic activity, some patients may complain of blurred vision, constipation, and dry mouth. Other complaints include dizziness, ataxia, and drowsiness.

419. The answer is D. *(Talbott, pp 836–841.)* In general, ECT is a relatively safe procedure. The morbidity and mortality are not significantly greater than for general anesthesia. The mortality is approximately one per 10,000 patients. Its principal indication is in the treatment of severe depression, particularly delusional depression and depression unresponsive to antidepressant medication. It is also used in elderly patients who cannot tolerate the side effects of antipsychotic or antidepressant agents. ECT has been found useful in the treatment of acute manic excitement that cannot be otherwise controlled. Impairment of memory is a common but variable complaint of patients receiving this treatment.

420–422. The answers are: 420-B, 421-C, 422-D. *(Kaplan, ed 4. pp 676–677.)* Lithium is the drug of choice for bipolar disorders. Its advantages over neuroleptics include a greater degree of specificity and ease in monitoring plasma levels, and it does not produce tardive dyskinesia. Therapeutic blood levels are from 0.8 to 1.2 mEq/L and it has a serum half-life of about 24 hours. Being a salt, it "competes" in the body with sodium and has effects on the heart, kidney, and thyroid. It can also cause birth defects. Unless indicated for another reason, a chest x-ray is not mandatory as a preadministration screen. Initial dosage is variable, but a test dose of 600 mg is very beneficial in establishing the regimen. The average adult is usually started at 600 mg three times a day.

423. The answer is D. *(Michels, vol 3, chap 45, pp 8–9.)* Double-blind crossover studies are done to control for individual differences in drug response and the placebo effect. They are conducted with neither the subject (patient) nor the researcher (physician) knowing whether the substance being taken is placebo or drug. This is double-blind. Crossover refers to changing from drug to placebo, or vice versa, in mid-study, again without knowledge of the subject or researcher.

424. The answer is D. *(Michels, vol 3, chap 45, pp 4–5.)* The half-life of a drug refers to how long it will take the body to metabolize one-half of the drug. Knowing the half-life is important in determining how often a drug should be administered. It is also helpful to know where a drug is metabolized. For example, drugs excreted via the renal system will be affected by any form of altered renal function. Organ pathology can greatly alter the normal half-life of a medication.

425. The answer is D. *(Michels, vol 2, chap 59, pp 12–13.)* The potency of an antipsychotic relates to its ability to block postsynaptic dopamine receptors. In general, the more potent the drug, the less sedating it is. Haldol is a high-potency neuroleptic, about sixty times more potent than Thorazine and Mellaril, and twenty times more potent than Navane and Stelazine.

426. The answer is D. *(Michels, vol 3, chap 50, pp 10–11.)* Tricyclic antidepressants inhibit the reuptake of serotonin and norepinephrine presynaptically. Recent research regarding tricyclics has discovered that up-and-down regulation of adrenergic receptor sensitivity is also important. The antipsychotic medications are a different class of substances. They are believed to exert their effects through blocking of postsynaptic dopamine receptors.

427. The answer is C. *(Michels, vol 3, chap 50, pp 11–13.)* Tricyclics, with their anticholinergic properties, can cause dry mouth, constipation, urinary retention, and orthostatic hypotension (a fall in blood pressure when sitting up). These side effects are commonly dose-related and subside to some extent with time in most patients.

Movement disorders are sometimes seen with use of antipsychotic drugs, but are not usually associated with tricyclics.

428. The answer is C. *(Kaplan, ed 4. p 652–656.)* Many drugs can produce disorientation as part of a toxic brain syndrome. However, the tricyclic antidepressants, such as amitriptyline, can stimulate psychosis in a schizophrenic patient or mania in a manic-depressive patient.

429. The answer is D. *(Michels, vol 2, chap 111, pp 2–5.)* Phenothiazines, tricyclic antidepressants, and antiparkinsonian agents (such as benztropine mesylate) all have anticholinergic properties. The action of these drugs becomes additive when they are administered in combination. It is not uncommon for persons receiving such a combination to show evidence of a mild organic brain syndrome, including difficulty in concentrating, impaired short-term memory, and disorientation, which often is more noticeable at night. Dry skin and palms are especially suggestive of atropinism.

430. The answer is B. *(Talbott, p 478.)* Several controlled studies have shown clomipramine, a tricyclic antidepressant, to be more effective in treating obsessive compulsive disorder than placebo or other active antidepressants. There is speculation that clomipramine's ability to potently block neuronal reuptake of serotonin may be involved in these effects. Whether clomipramine's effects are specifically antiobsessional, as opposed to antidepressant, is still a matter of controversy.

431. The answer is D. *(Michels, vol 3, chap 17, pp 7–8, 10.)* The minor tranquilizers or antianxiety agents, such as diazepam, are similar to barbiturates and other central nervous system depressants in that tolerance develops to both their sedating and their antianxiety effects. As a result, effectiveness diminishes with chronic administration.

432. The answer is C. *(Michels, vol 1, chap 61, p 19.)* The antimanic effect of lithium on manic patients usually is observed in 7 to 10 days. If a patient is agitated, sleepless, or otherwise unmanageable during the initiation of lithium therapy, an antipsychotic agent (either haloperidol or a phenothiazine) may be used.

433. The answer is D. *(Gilman, ed 7. p 403.)* Fluphenazine decanoate is the decanoic-acid ester of fluphenazine (Prolixin). Esterification of fluphenazine slows its release from the injection site. The duration of action of intramuscular fluphenazine decanoate averages 2 weeks, with a range of from 1 to 3 weeks.

434. The answer is C. *(Kaplan, ed 4. p 634.)* A number of controlled studies have demonstrated that chlorpromazine (Thorazine), when given in daily dosages of 300 mg or greater, was a significantly more effective antipsychotic agent than was placebo. At dosages below 300 mg, this effect was not demonstrated clearly, although other effects of chlorpromazine are noted at lower dosages.

435. The answer is B. *(Gilman, ed 7. pp 396–397.)* Antipsychotic drugs block dopamine receptor sites. Blockade of dopamine receptors in the limbic system is believed to be responsible for the antipsychotic effects. Blockage in the basal ganglia results in the "extrapyramidal" side effects of the drugs.

436. The answer is A. *(Gilman, ed 7. pp 137–138, 419–421.)* The anticholinergic or atropinic side effects of the tricyclic antidepressants can be pronounced. Dry mouth, for example, is routinely produced by therapeutic dosages of tricyclic antidepressant agents. Among the tricyclic antidepressants, amitriptyline is one of the most potent anticholinergic agents and desipramine the least. The anticholinergic effects of the phenothiazines are less strong. Lithium and the benzodiazepines are not atropinic.

437. The answer is D. *(Kaplan, ed 4. p 659.)* Severe reactions, even death, have been reported in persons receiving an MAO inhibitor who were given a high dose of imipramine. This observation has led to the belief that the two drugs are a lethal combination. Although the combination should not be used routinely, it currently is being investigated for use in patients who have refractory depression.

438. The answer is D. *(Gilman, ed 7, p 427.)* The only one of the major drugs used in psychiatry that does not produce some sedation or euphoria in normal subjects is lithium. This observation appears to be related to the clinical finding that persons receiving lithium therapy, unlike those taking phenothiazines or tricyclic antidepressants, seldom complain of feeling drugged.

439. The answer is C. *(Kaplan, ed 4. pp 150, 501, 774.)* Depression in elderly persons, especially those who already have some evidence of dementia, may suggest deterioration of the organic process. The differentiation of progressing dementia from depression may be impossible. If the onset of symptoms is reasonably abrupt (1 or 2 months) and the individual has other signs suggestive of depression (e.g., changes in sleeping and eating habits) accompanied by motor retardation or agitation, depression should be considered. It certainly is preferable to consider a trial of antidepressants, which might be beneficial, rather than to assume a person's dementia is progressive and untreatable.

440. The answer is B. *(Kaplan, ed 4. pp 1684–1690.)* Methylphenidate and the amphetamines, when effective, can lengthen attention span, reduce hyperactivity, and increase frustration tolerance in children who have attention deficit disorder. As a result, school performance improves, and the children become more sensitive to family and friends. Although school performance is improved by the increased attention span, affected children already may be considerably behind peers in academic achievement. Therefore, it is necessary to place these children in grades appropriate to their level of achievement, and if perceptual problems persist, they should be enrolled in special education classes.

441. The answer is C. *(Michels, vol 2, chap 89, p 8.)* Chlordiazepoxide (Librium) frequently is used in the treatment of persons in alcoholic withdrawal. Dosage must be sufficient to relieve tremors and agitation. Daily administration of more than 400 mg is seldom required.

442. The answer is C. *(Kaplan, ed 4. pp 829, 830.)* The therapeutic serum concentration of lithium for manic patients is 0.8 to 1.2 mEq/L. In maintenance therapy, a level of 0.8 to 1.0 mEq/L usually is sufficient. At lithium levels higher than 1.5 mEq/L, the incidence of side effects rapidly increases.

443. The answer is B. *(Kaplan, ed 4. pp 656–657.)* Cardiac arrhythmia, which sometimes can be fatal, is the most common dangerous consequence of an overdose of tricyclic antidepressant. For this reason, electrocardiographic monitoring is advised for persons who have taken a significant overdose. Physostigmine can be used to reverse the anticholinergic effects of the drug.

444. The answer is E. *(Kaplan, ed 4. p 824.)* Improvement in the condition of a depressed patient receiving a tricyclic antidepressant at an adequate dosage may be noted at the end of 1 week, is usually present by 2 weeks, but may not occur until the third week. For this reason, an adequate trial of a tricyclic antidepressant requires at least 3 weeks of treatment. Although patients who have a partial response may continue to improve, those who have not responded to treatment at the end of 3 weeks either require treatment at higher dosage or need different treatment.

445. The answer is C. *(Gilman, ed 7. pp 402–408.)* The antipsychotic drugs listed in the question are arranged in order of increasing extrapyramidal effects and decreasing anticholinergic, hypotensive, and sedative effects. Knowledge of the position of a drug along this side-effect gradient is useful in selecting the most suitable drug for a given individual. It should be remembered, too, that individuals experience a variety of side effects for which they exhibit variable tolerances.

446. The answer is D. *(Kaplan, ed 4. p 637.)* All the antipsychotic compounds currently in use are equal in their antipsychotic effects when used in the appropriate dosage. Dosage varies because the drugs vary in potency on a milligram per milligram basis. Therefore, the primary factor affecting the selection of an antipsychotic agent is its potential for causing side effects. Cost and antiemetic effects also vary among these drugs.

447. The answer is D. *(Kaplan, ed 4. pp 824, 825.)* The effective dosage range of imipramine for most patients is 75 to 300 mg daily. In a few persons, dosages above or below this range may be required because of unusual pharmacokinetics. A common error is to continue treatment at inadequate dosage levels.

448. The answer is B. *(Kaplan, ed 4. pp 632–637.)* Guanethidine (Ismelin) produces its antihypertensive effect after its uptake by peripheral noradrenergic neurons. Because tricyclic antidepressants block this uptake mechanism, guanethidine cannot reach its site of action.

449. The answer is B. *(Kaplan, ed 4. pp 1229–1230.)* Haloperidol has been reported to reduce symptoms by 90 percent in most people who have Gilles de la Tourette's syndrome. The dosage prescribed by clinicians ranges considerably, from 6 to 180 mg daily. Other antipsychotic drugs and minor tranquilizers have been shown to be less effective.

450. The answer is A. *(Talbott, pp 1135–1136.)* Although any sedating drug has the potential for adding to the confusion of an elderly person, the barbiturates are most frequently associated with paradoxical agitation or excitement. Chloral hydrate and flurazepam (Dalmane) are useful in treating insomnia in older persons. In the treatment of insomnia in an elderly patient who has either psychosis or depression, an antipsychotic or antidepressant drug may be indicated.

451. The answer is E. *(Kaplan, ed 4. p 885.)* Chlorpromazine, through its alpha-adrenergic blockade, blocks the alpha-stimulating effect of epinephrine, allowing the beta-stimulating effect to predominate. Thus, instead of having a pressor effect, epinephrine produces hypotension. Hypotension in a person receiving chlorpromazine should be treated with volume expansion and administration of norepinephrine, which has alpha-stimulating but not beta-stimulating effects.

452. The answer is B (1, 3). *(Talbott, p 433.)* The syndrome of seasonal affective disorder often presents with the regular occurrence of major depressive episodes in the late fall or winter, with remission in the spring. Sometimes hypomania will appear in the summer. Patients are often treated with antidepressant medication, but tend to be poor responders. Exposure to several hours of bright artificial light (phototherapy) brings rapid and marked improvement to the majority of patients suffering from this syndrome.

453. The answer is E (all). *(Kaplan, ed 4. p 1492.)* Schizophrenia is a chronic psychotic disorder. It is heterogeneous with diverse pharmacologic treatments. The mainstay of treatment for schizophrenia is the group of medications called antipsychotics or neuroleptics. They include the phenothiazines (Thorazine, Mellaril, Stelazine, Prolixin), butyrophenones (Haldol), thioxanthenes (Navane), and others.

Lithium is the treatment of choice in mania, but has also been shown to be effective in the treatment of other psychotic illnesses.

454. The answer is B (1, 3). *(Kaplan, ed 4. pp 386–387.)* Opium is produced from the seeds of poppy plants. The dried exudate of the unripe seeds is powdered to produce alkaloids. The ones used in clinical medicine include morphine, codeine, thebaine, papaverine, and noscapine. The morphine content of opium is 10 percent. These drugs are potent analgesics with strong addictive potentials. Thorazine and diazepam are synthetic compounds, thorazine being an antipsychotic and diazepam a muscle relaxant, anticonvulsant, and anxiolytic.

455. The answer is A (1, 2, 3). *(Kaplan, ed 4. pp 643–646.)* Extrapyramidal reactions during the first weeks of chlorpromazine treatment generally are divided into three categories. Acute dystonic reactions, the first category, often occur within the first few days of treatment and respond dramatically to antiparkinsonian drugs. Akathisia (motor restlessness), the second type of extrapyramidal reaction, may be difficult to differentiate from a worsening of the underlying psychosis; however, unlike the latter, akathisia usually will respond to a reduction in the dosage of the antipsychotic agent. Parkinsonian syndrome is the third category of early extrapyramidal reactions. Tardive dyskinesia is an extrapyramidal syndrome that results from chronic use of antipsychotic medication over a period of years.

456. The answer is C (2, 4). *(Kaplan, ed 4. p 641.)* Dry mouth, blurred vision, and constipation are common dose-dependent anticholinergic side effects of chlorpromazine. Administration of an anticholinergic, antiparkinsonian drug will exacerbate these symptoms. The presence of difficulty in initiating urination, which is another anticholinergic side effect, should be ascertained, because it can lead to urinary retention.

457. The answer is C (2, 4). *(Michels, vol 1, chap 55, p 26.)* The woman described has a parkinsonian syndrome, symptoms of which include rigidity, tremor, hypokinesia, and micrographia. In addition, she is more likely to have a masked expression or a lack of affect than euphoria. Corneal opacities, which are late in onset and are relatively uncommon side effects of the use of phenothiazines, are unrelated to the parkinsonian syndrome.

458. The answer is C (2, 4). *(Kaplan, ed 4. pp 1491–1492.)* Most studies of plasma levels of antipsychotics have failed to document a clear relation between drug level and clinical efficacy. Attempts to establish such a relation are complicated by the fact that many antipsychotics, such as chlorpromazine, have metabolites that also possess antipsychotic effects. There is no clear evidence that plasma levels predict which patients will develop extrapyramidal or other side effects.

459. The answer is B (1, 3). *(Michels, vol 2, chap 89, p 8.)* Benzodiazepines demonstrate some cross-tolerance with other central nervous system depressants, including alcohol, barbiturates, and nonbarbiturate hypnotics, such as glutethimide (Doriden) and methyprylon (Noludar). This cross-tolerance not only enables chlordiazepoxide to be substituted for alcohol in the treatment of alcohol withdrawal but also explains the potential for benzodiazepine abuse by people who have previously abused other central nervous system depressants.

460. The answer is D (4). *(Kaplan, ed 4. pp 478–479.)* The benzodiazepines are more effective than placebo in the treatment of anxiety. Their antianxiety effect is more noticeable in persons who have chronic anxiety, for whom there is a low placebo response, than in persons who have acute anxiety; this latter group responds well to both active drug and placebo. Comparative studies suggest that meprobamate (Equanil, Miltown) clearly is not superior to benzodiazepines. For anxiety that is part of a more specific disorder, such as schizophrenia, treatment should be directed at the underlying disorder.

461. The answer is B (1, 3). *(Kaplan, ed 4. p 824. Schatzberg, pp 29–57.)* Maprotiline (Ludiomil), although similar to the tricyclics, belongs to the tetracyclic class. Trazodone (Desyrel), a triazolopyridine, has a structure that is completely unrelated to the tricyclics. Protriptyline (Vivactil) and doxepin (Sinequan) are secondary and tertiary amine tricyclics, respectively.

462. The answer is B (1, 3). *(Michels, vol 2, chap 59, pp 10–11.)* Side effects occurring during the initiation of lithium therapy include nausea, vomiting, and diarrhea. Appearance of these symptoms usually occurs at the peak plasma level. Hand tremor is one of the most common side effects during maintenance treatment and may improve with low-dose propranolol.

463. The answer is C (2, 4). *(Gilman, ed 7. p 399.)* The phenothiazines have a number of endocrine effects. Galactorrhea or amenorrhea can result from the drugs' effects on prolactin and gonadotropins. Phenothiazines also reduce secretion of growth hormone and adrenocorticotropin. Weight gain is a common side effect of the use of phenothiazines.

464. The answer is C (2, 4). *(Kaplan, ed 4. pp 584, 1502, 1506.)* Nausea, vomiting, headaches, muscular discomfort, insomnia, and anxiety have been reported to follow abrupt withdrawal of phenothiazines. Although they may produce the symptoms of physical dependence that are listed above, phenothiazines are not considered to be addictive, because their withdrawal does not lead to craving. Withdrawal is not associated with convulsions.

465. The answer is B (1, 3). *(Kaplan, ed 4. pp 721–722.)* The long-term risk of tardive dyskinesia can be reduced by restricting the use of antipsychotic drugs to those individuals who require chronic antipsychotic treatment—primarily, individuals with recurrent psychosis. Chronic administration should be avoided in syndromes such as chronic anxiety in which other treatment could be employed. Individuals needing chronic antipsychotic drug therapy require careful observation, because the tardive dyskinesia syndrome may more likely be reversible if it is detected early and the antipsychotic agent discontinued promptly. Antiparkinsonian drugs play no role in the treatment of tardive dyskinesia; in fact, their use may worsen the syndrome.

466. The answer is B (1, 3). *(Gilman, ed 7. pp 434–435, 437, 470. Kaplan, ed 4. pp 96, 136–137, 1322.)* Diazepam is the treatment of choice for persons in status epilepticus and is effective in a high percentage of cases. Because it can reduce or eliminate stage-4 sleep, it is used to treat persons suffering from night terrors. In addition to its sedating action, diazepam can be used as a hypnotic. Although diazepam is used as a muscle relaxant, benzodiazepines have not been proved more effective in producing muscle relaxation than either placebo or aspirin. Some muscle relaxation may result with use of any central nervous system depressant.

467. The answer is D (4). *(Kaplan, ed 4. pp 263–264.)* Several double-blind studies have demonstrated the superiority of lithium over placebo in the treatment of mania. Although there have been interest in and suggestive evidence for the usefulness of lithium in the treatment of bipolar depression, its antidepressant effect in major depression has not been fully established. Lithium is not used in the treatment of patients who have a schizophrenic psychosis or anxiety.

468. The answer is B (1, 3). *(Kaplan, ed 4. pp 831–832.)* Because lithium is excreted primarily by the kidney, limited renal function, as indicated by a very low creatinine clearance, may be a contraindication to lithium therapy. If sodium intake is reduced significantly, lithium excretion drops and lithium intoxication can result. Lithium often is used in combination with other psychotropic drugs for the treatment of acute mania or the depressed phase of a bipolar disorder.

469. The answer is B (1, 3). *(Kaplan, ed 4. pp 654–655.)* The tricyclic antidepressants produce a number of side effects, including dry mouth, loss of the accommodation reflex, postural hypotension, tachycardia, and constipation. These side effects are annoying but usually tolerable. Urinary retention and paralytic ileus are two side effects that are much less common but much more serious.

470. The answer is D (4). *(Kaplan, ed 4. pp 650–657.)* Tricyclic antidepressants reduce depression in persons who have primary depressive illness. In normal subjects, tricyclics act neither as euphoriants nor as stimulants; as a result, they appear to have a "corrective" action in the treatment of primary depressive illness. Tricyclic antidepressants are not effective in the treatment of mania and may, in fact, exacerbate a manic syndrome. They also do not appear to be effective in treating the depressed mood of demoralized persons.

471. The answer is C (2, 4). *(Hales, p 68.)* The action of reserpine has been important in the development of the amine hypothesis of depression. Reserpine, which is known to produce depression in certain individuals, depletes nerve endings of stored norepinephrine and serotonin. It was hypothesized that a reduction of these neurotransmitters is related to the onset of depression.

472. The answer is C (2, 4). *(Kaplan, ed 4. p 327.)* Imipramine reduces the frequency and severity of panic attacks in patients who have panic disorder. Imipramine therapy has been reported to be beneficial for those with obsessive compulsive personality disorder. It may exacerbate mania or psychosis.

473. The answer is C (2, 4). *(Michels, vol 1, chap 61, p 20.)* Early signs of lithium toxicity include confusion, lethargy, coarse tremor, dysarthria, vomiting, diarrhea, and ataxia. If these signs appear, lithium should be discontinued immediately so that the plasma level can decrease. Continuation of lithium treatment can lead to hyperreflexia, muscle tremor and fasciculation, seizures, coma, and sometimes death.

474. The answer is A (1, 2, 3). *(Kaplan, ed 4. pp 26–27.)* Most people rapidly develop tolerance to sedation and accommodate to the lightheadedness associated with the hypotensive side effects of phenothiazines. Tolerance to extrapyramidal side effects, which develops within 2 or 3 months, allows antiparkinsonian agents to be discontinued in many cases. Because patients do not develop a tolerance to the phenothiazines' antipsychotic action, these drugs can be used for years in maintenance therapy.

475. The answer is C (2, 4). *(Kaplan, ed 4. pp 826–828.)* Major adverse reactions, which interrupt treatment, are more frequent in patients over 60 years of age and in patients concurrently receiving antipsychotic drugs with the tricyclic. The antipsychotic-tricyclic combination is especially associated with increased "anticholinergic" side effects, which may be mediated by central rather than peripheral mechanisms. Plasma concentrations of these drugs are not routinely elevated in patients having serious side effects.

476. The answer is B (1, 3). *(Kaplan, ed 4. pp 641–643.)* Tardive dyskinesia is a syndrome usually occurring late in the course of treatment with antipsychotic drugs. It is characterized most commonly by repetitive sucking or smacking movements of the mouth or repetitive movements of the tongue. Less commonly, affected persons exhibit choreiform movements of the limbs and athetoid twisting of the trunk. Though the syndrome is not medically dangerous, it is disfiguring and may interfere severely with functioning. In some persons, tardive dyskinesia is irreversible.

Law and Ethics in Psychiatry

DIRECTIONS: Each question below contains five suggested responses. Select the **one best** response to each question.

477. When a subpoena is delivered ordering release of psychiatric records, the psychiatrist

(A) must release the records immediately
(B) may update and modify the records before releasing them
(C) may demand a judicial hearing before releasing them
(D) may release them only with the patient's permission
(E) may refuse to release them because of doctor-patient privilege

478. All states now have laws requiring the physician to report cases of

(A) heroin abuse
(B) drug addicts admitted to hospitals
(C) psychosis with hallucinations ordering violence
(D) child abuse
(E) pedophilia

479. When a patient's illness has resulted in an inability to understand and therefore manage personal or financial affairs, a guardian may be designated after the patient is declared incompetent by

(A) a family member with power of attorney
(B) a judge following a hearing
(C) a psychiatrist, after a thorough examination of mental status
(D) a spouse
(E) a hospital administrator upon the advice of a psychiatrist

480. The standard for criminal responsibility in most U.S. federal courts is the

(A) product rule
(B) M'Naghten rule
(C) American Law Institute test
(D) irresistible impulse test
(E) Currens test

481. Privileged communication means

(A) that psychiatrists have the privilege of disclosing information about a patient to other psychiatrists or physicians

(B) that the information revealed by psychiatrists at a probate hearing is handled as privileged

(C) that psychiatrists are granted by the court the "privilege" to disclose information about a specific patient

(D) that patients have the statutory right to prevent psychiatrists from disclosing confidential information

(E) none of the above

482. In the nineteenth century, due-process procedures for civilly committed patients were expanded as the result of the work and writings of

(A) Dorothea Dix
(B) Elizabeth Packard
(C) Lyman Beecher
(D) William Lloyd Garrison
(E) Isaac Ray

483. The landmark decision in *Tarasoff v. Regents of California* held that a therapist has

(A) an obligation to protect the confidentiality of information obtained during therapy

(B) an obligation to warn the university when students are involved in any illegal activities

(C) an obligation to report to university authorities the presence of a student who is involved in illegal drug sales

(D) an obligation to warn the potential victim of a potentially violent patient

(E) an obligation to give informed consent to patients of the student health center who are given neuroleptic medications

DIRECTIONS: Each question below contains four suggested responses of which **one or more** is correct. Select

A	if	**1, 2, and 3**	are correct
B	if	**1 and 3**	are correct
C	if	**2 and 4**	are correct
D	if	**4**	is correct
E	if	**1, 2, 3, and 4**	are correct

484. The physician is not legally or ethically bound to continue treatment if

(1) dismissed by a patient who is believed competent
(2) the patient is given ample medication to last until he or she finds a new therapist
(3) there is suitable notice and assistance given to find a substitute therapist
(4) the patient is uncooperative with the treatment

485. The ethical issue underlying the principle of informed consent centers on whether or not the patient has *knowingly* consented. Essential elements of informed consent include

(1) the patient's competency
(2) the patient's ability to rationally understand
(3) the patient's knowledge of the circumstances of the treatment or research
(4) voluntary agreement without coercion

486. The principles of informed consent and the usual common-law elements of disclosure include

(1) the nature of the procedure or treatment
(2) the risks that are material, substantial, probable, or significant
(3) the anticipated benefits including probability of success
(4) the alternatives

487. Informed consent need *not* be obtained from

(1) patients involved in emergencies that threaten life or serious bodily harm
(2) patients legally committed to a mental hospital
(3) patients who waive decision-making and information disclosure
(4) patients who are clearly and manifestly psychotic

488. Tarasoff II, the second decision by the California Supreme Court, revised the original ruling by

(1) requiring the warning of only "identifiable" victims
(2) declaring immunity for the police
(3) requiring hospitalization of patients deemed dangerous
(4) finding a duty to protect victims, not just warn them

489. In 1843 Daniel M'Naghten was tried and found not guilty by reason of insanity. This insanity verdict resulted in the

(1) establishment of the "good versus evil" standard
(2) development of standards used by many states
(3) establishment of delusions as the *sine qua non* of legal insanity
(4) lifelong confinement of M'Naghten in an asylum

490. Correct statements about the use of hypnosis to "refresh" the memory of witnesses and victims include which of the following?

(1) It is likely to be more accurate if the hypnotist guides the imagery on the basis of prior reports
(2) It is best used just prior to testifying
(3) It does not alter the subjective certainty of an identification
(4) It may produce confabulations that are recalled as "real"

491. Physicians have the duty to disclose risks of treatment to their patients EXCEPT in instances where

(1) minimal risks are involved
(2) a medical emergency is involved
(3) disclosure would definitively result in the deterioration of a patient's physical or mental condition
(4) disclosure might cause the patient to refuse treatment

492. Competence to stand trial is described by which of the following statements?

(1) The U.S. Supreme Court has not yet defined a standard
(2) It is possible for a defendant to be competent for one charge and not for another
(3) Mental status must be assessed both at the time of the crime and at the time of trial
(4) A person with a total organic amnesia for the events of a crime still may be judged competent

493. Psychiatrists who have sexual relationships with their patients are

(1) in violation of the American Psychiatric Association's guidelines for ethical conduct
(2) liable to malpractice suits, even if the patient consented
(3) in jeopardy of having their license revoked by their state medical licensing board
(4) liable to prosecution for rape

494. Psychiatrists giving testimony in court should know that

(1) their testimony must conform to the "reasonable medical certainty" standard
(2) they may give opinion testimony if accepted as an expert witness
(3) they may give opinion as to the ultimate issue to be decided by the trier of fact
(4) they may not use lie detectors or other such tests, which are inadmissible, to support an opinion

495. Psychiatrists often are called upon to evaluate testamentary capacity. Essential components of a valid will include

(1) knowledge of the nature and extent of one's assets
(2) knowledge of relatives and natural heirs
(3) knowledge that a will is being made
(4) freedom from undue influence

DIRECTIONS: The group of questions below consists of lettered headings followed by a set of numbered items. For each numbered item select the **one** lettered heading with which it is **most** closely associated. Each lettered heading may be used **once, more than once, or not at all.**

Questions 496–500

Match the following.
(A) M'Naghten rule
(B) Irresistible impulse rule
(C) American Law Institute: Model Penal Code
(D) Durham rule
(E) *Mens rea* elements

496. Psychiatric testimony should only be addressed to the issue of state of mind and criminal intent at the time of the crime

497. An insanity defense related to inability to know the nature and quality of the act being done, or that what was being done was wrong

498. An accused is not criminally responsible if the unlawful act was the product of mental disease or mental defect

499. A test of criminal responsibility that specifically excludes those conditions that may have associated sociopathic behaviors, such as some personality disorders

500. "A person is not responsible for criminal conduct if at the time of such conduct as a result of mental disease or defect he lacks substantial capacity either to appreciate the criminality (wrongfulness) of his conduct or to conform his conduct to the requirements of the law"

Law and Ethics in Psychiatry
Answers

477. The answer is C. *(Michels, vol 3, chap 31, pp 9–10.)* A subpoena does not require that the psychiatrist immediately surrender the psychiatric records. It cannot be enforced until there is an opportunity to appear before a judge in a hearing. This offers an opportunity to present arguments such as belief that the release of the information will be destructive to the patient or the family. By contrast, a court-approved search warrant by law enforcement officers does not provide such an opportunity for challenge.

478. The answer is D. *(Michels, vol 3, chap 31, pp 13–16.)* Respect for the patient's confidentiality is considered by all psychiatrists to be essential for effective clinical practice. Psychiatrists have traditionally resisted attempts to place them in the role of an informer. The American Medical Association and the American Psychiatric Association have endorsed an additional ethical obligation to society under certain circumstances. All states now have laws for reporting of child abuse. Some states, but not all, require that users of certain drugs be reported as well as persons believed likely to commit violence. There are also jurisdictions that protect the confidentiality of addicts and drug-dependent persons voluntarily seeking treatment. There is no obligation to report the existence of a sexual disorder that might result in unlawful acts.

479. The answer is B. *(Michels, vol 3, chap 31, p 12.)* Guardianship can only be established by a judicial proceeding, and careful attention is given to assuring the patient's rights. The psychiatrist may be called upon to give testimony regarding competency, but only the court can appoint someone to make decisions on the patient's behalf.

480. The answer is C. *(Halleck, pp 214–224. Kaplan, ed 4. p 1967.)* Most U.S. federal courts presently use the American Law Institute (ALI) test, or a minor variation, to determine criminal responsibility. The ALI standard states, "It shall be a defense that the defendant at the time of the proscribed conduct, as a result of mental disease or defect lacked substantial capacity either to appreciate the wrongfulness of his conduct or to conform his conduct to the requirements of the law." Many jurisdictions have appended a section that states, "The terms mental disease or defect do not include an abnormality manifested only by repeated criminal or otherwise antisocial conduct." This provision is designed to prevent persons with antisocial personality from offering an insanity defense. Recent decisions in some jurisdictions suggest that the federal judiciary may be moving back toward M'Naghten.

481. The answer is D. *(Kaplan, ed 4. pp 1963–1965.)* Privileged communication must be provided by statute. Where the privilege exists, it is essentially "owned" by the person whose medical information is being sought. Individuals may waive the privilege and allow their psychiatrists to testify. Because there are many qualifications to statutory privilege, some feel that the concept is almost meaningless.

482. The answer is B. *(Kaplan, ed 4. pp 1978–1979.)* In 1860, Elizabeth Packard was confined involuntarily in accordance with an Illinois statute permitting commitment of a married woman on the petition of her husband "without the evidence of insanity or distraction usually required in other cases." Following her release and attempted reconfinement, Mrs. Packard went on a crusade against civil commitment, and her book *Modern Persecution, or Insane Hospitals Unveiled* resulted in the revision of commitment statutes in many states. Jury trials often were mandated as a due-process requirement. However, by the beginning of the twentieth century many of these revised statutes had been repealed. In the 1960s, there was a resurgence of attention concerning the civil rights and abuse of state hospital patients, which has resulted in the current revision of commitment statutes, including greater legal safeguards for persons facing commitment.

483. The answer is D. *(Michels, vol 3, chap 31, pp 13–15.)* The Tarasoff decision was a landmark case in determining that psychotherapists have an obligation to warn third parties who are in danger. In this instance, the therapist had an obligation to warn the potential victim of a student who had threatened to kill the girl who had rejected him. He ultimately killed her, and thus began the litigation.

484. The answer is B (1, 3). *(Michels, vol 3, chap 29, pp 7–8.)* There is no legal obligation to accept any patient for therapy, but once the doctor-patient relationship is established there are legal and ethical obligations on the doctor to keep properly informed about the patient's condition and to provide for psychiatric needs. Abandonment that results in injury may establish grounds for malpractice. The safety and welfare of the patient is paramount. There is an obligation to offer assistance in finding alternative treatment. To simply provide medication does not take into account that the patient may decompensate and injure himself during the period it takes to do this. The therapist might terminate treatment with an uncooperative patient, but only if assistance is given in finding a new therapist.

485. The answer is E (all). *(Talbott, p 1089.)* Issues of informed consent arise whenever any treatment is to be initiated, as well as when there is possible participation in a research study. The ethical issue of "knowing consent" requires that the patient be competent and capable of rationally understanding the relevant issues. The circumstances of the treatment or research must be fully explained, and the patient must voluntarily agree. There must not be coercion or improper inducement. The ethical requirements become particularly important, and difficult, when dealing with psychotic or organically impaired patients whose capacity to evaluate the issues may be clouded.

486. The answer is E (all). *(Michels, vol 3, chap 30, pp 2–7.)* Informed consent is a matter of both ethics and law. It reflects respect for the patient's autonomy as a person who can reason and make decisions regarding personal welfare. The courts have upheld these principles, and it is important that physicians know the legal rules that govern disclosure in their state. Federal grants in support of research carry very explicit requirements regarding informed consent.

487. The answer is B (1, 3). *(Halleck, pp 89–96. Michels, vol 3, chap 30, pp 6–7.)* While there are many legal debates about just what constitutes an emergency, the courts have generally held that emergencies that threaten life or serious harm to self or others constitute an exception to the requirements for informed consent. Most courts have also rejected the idea that commitment and incompetency are synonymous, and of course not all manifestly psychotic patients are incompetent. The physician need not give information to those patients who waive their rights, but the waiver should be clearly documented in the record.

488. The answer is C (2, 4). *(Michels, vol 3, chap 31, pp 14–16.)* Tarasoff I held that psychotherapists and the police have a duty to warn third parties who are in danger. Tarasoff II stated that once a therapist determines or reasonably should have determined that a patient poses a serious danger of violence to others, he "bears a duty to exercise reasonable care to protect the foreseeable victim of that danger." This is an expansion of the more narrow duty to warn. It leaves unclear what actions would be legally sufficient. The decision also eliminated the police from liability. In 1980 in *Thompson v. County of Alameda* (614 P.2d 728) the California Supreme Court suggested that a "precondition to liability" is an intended victim who is "readily identifiable." Other jurisdictions have gone beyond California and held that an expanded duty exists to groups or categories of potential victims (*Lipari v. Sears, Roebuck & Co.,* 497 Fed Supp. 185 [1980]; *Petersen v. State,* 671 P.2d 230 [1983]).

489. The answer is C (2, 4). *(Kaplan, ed 4. pp 1965–1970.)* Following the insanity verdict in M'Naghten's case, the outraged Queen and House of Lords demanded from the judges a standard for criminal responsibility. This standard, which did not affect M'Naghten's case, stated that "it must be clearly proved that at the time of the commiting of the act, the party accused was labouring under such a defect of reason, from disease of the mind, as not to know the nature and quality of the act he was doing; or if he did know it, that he did not know that he was doing what was wrong." The defense relied heavily on the ideas of the American psychiatrist

Isaac Ray, whose historic work, *A Treatist on the Medical Jurisprudence of Insanity,* was published in 1837. M'Naghten was detained in an asylum for his remaining 22 years. Recently release of those found not guilty by reason of insanity has occurred more rapidly, and a number of states now place the burden of proof on the state to show the need for continued confinement.

490. The answer is D (4). *(Talbott, pp 916–917.)* Hypnosis can systematically bias a witness, especially if the hypnotist has preconceptions about the "facts" of a case. Preconceptions and cues offered by the hypnotist may cause confabulation and the production of pseudomemories, which are recalled as "real." These false memories can be "recalled" with a heightened sense of conviction and certainty, which further invalidates the testimony. Hypnosis is best used to provide useful leads that can be independently confirmed. Following hypnosis, memory may be irretrievably altered. Truthfulness cannot be ascertained by hypnosis even in deeply hypnotizable subjects; both malingering and lying can occur during hypnosis.

491. The answer is A (1, 2, 3). *(Kaplan, ed 4. pp 1981–1984.)* There are a number of exceptions to the informed consent doctrine. Physicians have a duty to disclose all significant or material risks. They must disclose alternative treatments. Medical emergencies (e.g., when a person is unconscious or otherwise incapable of consenting) have long been accepted as exceptions under the doctrine of implied consent. Courts have also recognized that a person's mental and emotional condition must be taken into account and that discretion must be employed in the manner and style of disclosing information. While there is a degree of latitude for the physician, it is better to err on the side of disclosure. The possibility that disclosure might prompt a person to forego treatment is not sufficient grounds for withholding information.

492. The answer is C (2, 4). *(Kaplan, ed 4. pp 1970–1972.)* In establishing a standard for competency of a defendant to stand trial, the U.S. Supreme Court (*Dusky v. United States,* 1960) said that the defendant must have "sufficient present ability to consult with his lawyer with a reasonable degree of rational understanding" and must have "a rational as well as factual understanding of the proceedings against him." The standard is variable in its interpretation, so that a person could be sufficiently rational to be deemed competent to stand trial for trespassing yet incompetent for a complicated murder or embezzlement charge. Competency to stand trial has nothing to do with the defendant's state of mind at the time of the alleged crime. An accused person's claim of being unable to remember or reconstruct events has met with little sympathetic response from the courts; because amnesia is not objectively verifiable, judges fear this condition could become "pandemic" if it were accepted as a standard for incompetence.

493. The answer is E (all). *(Talbott, pp 1087–1088).* In "The Principles of Medical Ethics with Annotations Especially Applicable to Psychiatry" the American

Psychiatric Association unequivocally states that sexual activity with patients is unethical. The intensity of the therapeutic relationship may activate sexual feelings and fantasies in both patient and therapist; sexual activity has been considered a dramatic example of the misuse and exploitation of the transference relationship. Psychiatrists have been prosecuted for rape in a few situations, and this approach has been advocated by Masters and Johnson. The number of malpractice suits has been increasing, with substantial settlements and subsequent loss of licensure. Peer review mechanisms have been of little help in controlling this problem.

494. The answer is A (1, 2, 3). *(Kaplan, ed 4. pp 1960–1965.)* In contrast to other witnesses, expert witnesses may give opinion testimony if they qualify as an expert in the area under consideration. Psychiatrists may give opinions regarding ultimate issues, such as competence or insanity. They also may use a variety of tests as a basis for their opinion. In situations in which legally inadmissible tests are used, the jury is instructed to weigh that evidence only for evaluating the credibility of the expert's opinion and not for the accuracy of the test. Clear and convincing evidence, preponderance of the evidence, and proof beyond a reasonable doubt all are legal standards of proof that judges and juries must use in decision-making. Expert medical testimony must conform to a "reasonable medical certainty" standard.

495. The answer is E (all). *(Kaplan, ed 4. pp 1976–1977.)* Although people have the authority to bequeath their estates to any persons or institution of their choice, they must have testamentary capacity—that is, knowledge of who their relatives are and who may have claim to their estate; a reasonable estimate of the extent of their assets; an awareness that they are signing a will; and an understanding of what is meant by a will. Undue influence may be grounds for invalidating part or all of a will, if it can be shown that the influence was sufficient to lead the testator to make a decision that otherwise would not have been made. Undue influence relates to voluntariness, rather than to cognitive capacity, and is a distinct and an important concept in evaluating a will.

496–500. The answers are: 496-E, 497-A, 498-D, 499-C, 500-C. *(Halleck, 214–219. Michels, vol 3, chap 27, pp 6–9.)* The AMA has recommended, and some states have codified, that the insanity defense be abolished. There is considerable question as to whether this can be done constitutionally. Such attempts often direct that the psychiatrist should only testify as to the *mens rea* elements in criminal trials. This is testimony that addresses the issue of whether the defendant possessed a criminal intent or state of mind at the time of the crime.

In 1843 Daniel M'Naghten was accused of killing the secretary of the Prime Minister of Great Britain. He was acquitted on grounds of insanity, and public outrage led to the development of the M'Naghten test regarding criminal insanity. It is a test primarily related to cognitive functions. It became the test of insanity in many jurisdictions in the United States and is still retained by some states.

The Durham rule, a 1954 decision by the District of Columbia Circuit Court, eliminated the cognitive issues that were associated with the M'Naghten rule, as well as the concept of irresistible impulse that had expanded it in some jurisdictions in order to introduce the concept of volitional control over one's behavior. It gave wide latitude to psychiatric testimony. It was rejected in 1972 because there was simply too much variation in psychiatric opinion as to what constituted the "product of mental disease or mental defect."

The Model Penal Code developed by the American Law Institute (ALI) did not attempt to define mental disease or defect, but it did specify that "the terms 'mental disease' or 'defect' do not include an abnormality manifested only by repeated criminal or otherwise antisocial conduct." This reflected the opinion that sociopaths should not be able to evade criminal responsibility for their acts by claiming that their behavior was on the basis of their psychiatric problem.

Most federal circuit courts and approximately 25 states have adopted at least parts of the rule developed by the ALI. The rule has at least some elements of cognitive (M'Naghten) and volitional (irresistible impulse) determinations. However, it is no longer an issue of "all or nothing." The word "appreciate," for example, acknowledges that a psychotic person may "know" right from wrong, but may lack an ability to truly comprehend the substance and consequences of the behavior. Consider the case of a psychotic who knows that murder is morally and legally wrong, but who kills a neighbor while acting under the influence of paranoid delusions and compelling hallucinations.

Bibliography

American Psychiatric Association: *Diagnostic and Statistical Manual of Mental Disorders,* 3rd ed., rev. *(DSM III-R).* Washington, American Psychiatric Association, 1987.

Bassuk EL, Birk AW (eds): *Emergency Psychiatry: Concepts, Methods, and Practices.* New York, Plenum Publishing, 1984.

Colarusso CA, Nemiroff RA: *Adult Development: A New Dimension in Psychodynamic Theory and Practice.* New York, Plenum Publishing, 1981.

Gilman AG, et al (eds): *Goodman and Gilman's The Pharmacological Basis of Therapeutics,* 7th ed. New York, Macmillan, 1985.

Hales RE, Yudofsky SC (eds): *American Psychiatric Press Textbook of Neuropsychiatry.* Washington, American Psychiatric Press, 1987.

Halleck S: *Law in the Practice of Psychiatry: A Handbook for Clinicians.* New York, Plenum Publishing, 1980.

Kaplan HI, Sadock BJ: *Comprehensive Textbook of Psychiatry,* 4th ed. Baltimore, Williams & Wilkins, 1984.

Michels R, Cavenar JO Jr (eds): *Psychiatry,* 3 vols. New York, Basic Books, 1985.

Nemeroff CB, Youngblood WW, Manberg PJ, et al: Regional brain concentrations of neuropeptides in Huntington's chorea and schizophrenia. *Science* 221:972–973, 1983.

Nicholi, AM Jr (ed): *The New Harvard Guide to Psychiatry.* Cambridge, Harvard University Press, Belknap Press, 1988.

Schatzberg AF, Cole JO: *Manual of Clinical Psychopharmacology.* Washington, American Psychiatric Press, 1986.

Stoudemire A, Fogel BS (eds): *Principles of Medical Psychiatry.* Orlando, Grune & Stratton, 1987.

Strauss JS, Carpenter WT Jr: *Schizophrenia.* New York, Plenum Publishing, 1981.

Talbott JA, Hales RE, Yudofsky SC (eds): *American Psychiatric Press Textbook of Psychiatry.* Washington, American Psychiatric Press, 1988.

Whybrow PC, Akiskal HS, McKinney WT Jr: *Mood Disorders: Toward a New Psychobiology.* New York, Plenum Publishing, 1984.